I0106366

This publication is intended to provide educational information for the reader on the covered subjects. It is not intended to take the place of personalized medical counseling, diagnosis, and treatment from a trained healthcare professional.

ISBN 978-1-998740-15-4 (Paperback)
ISBN 978-1-998740-16-1 (eBook)

Printed and bound in USA
Published by Loons Press

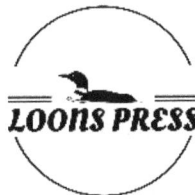

LOONS PRESS

Table Of Contents

How To Overcome OCD

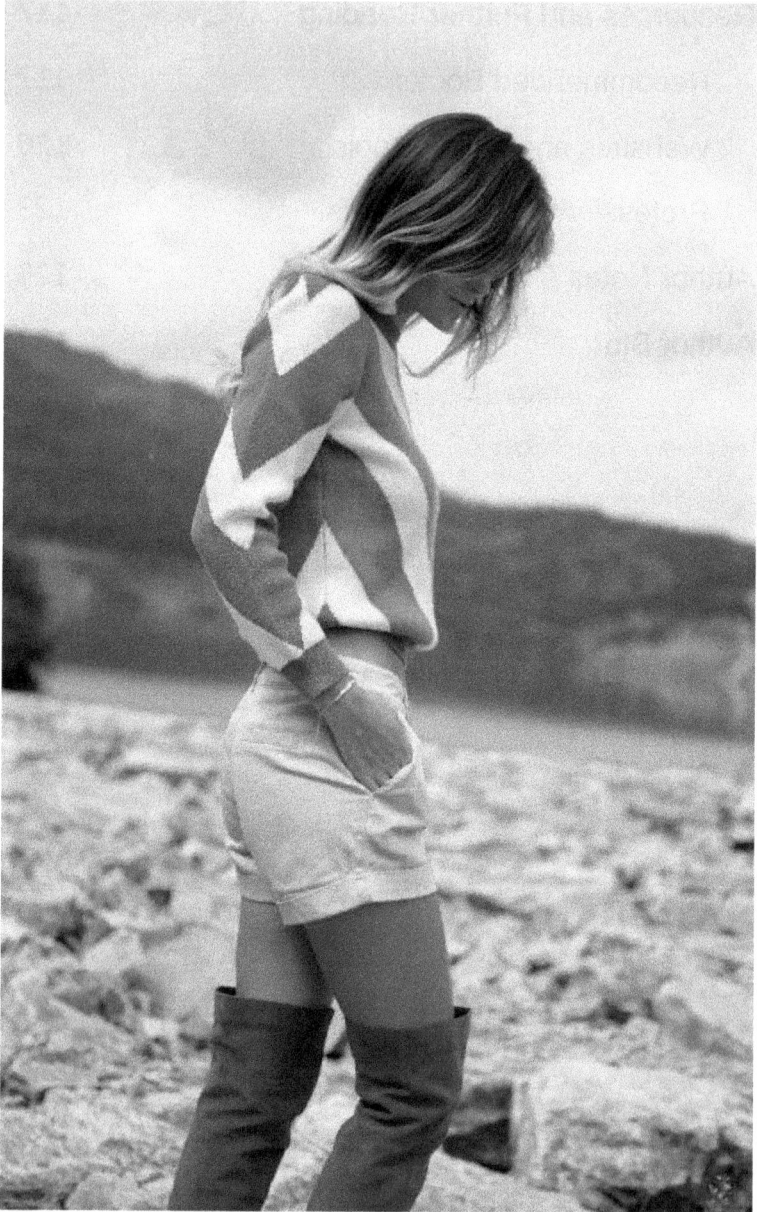

Chapter 1
Understanding OCD

Definition and Symptoms

Obsessive-Compulsive Disorder (OCD) is a mental health condition characterized by persistent, unwanted thoughts (obsessions) and repetitive behaviors or mental acts (compulsions) that a person feels driven to perform. These obsessions can provoke significant anxiety, leading individuals to engage in compulsive behaviors in an attempt to alleviate their distress.

The cycle of obsession and compulsion can become debilitating, impacting daily functioning, relationships, and overall quality of life. Understanding the definition of OCD is crucial for recognizing its symptoms and seeking appropriate help.

Common symptoms of OCD include intrusive thoughts about harm, cleanliness, or orderliness, which can manifest in various ways. For instance, individuals may experience fears related to contamination, leading them to wash their hands excessively or avoid certain environments. Similarly, doubts about safety can prompt repetitive checking behaviors, such as ensuring doors are locked or appliances are turned off. These obsessions are not just fleeting thoughts; they are persistent and can occupy a significant portion of a person's daily life.

Compulsions are the actions taken in response to these obsessions, often intended to neutralize anxiety or prevent a feared event from happening. While these behaviors may provide temporary relief, they do not address the root of the anxiety and can reinforce the cycle of OCD. Common compulsions include counting, arranging items in a specific order, or repeating certain phrases. Individuals may recognize that their compulsions are irrational, yet the overwhelming anxiety from the obsessions compels them to continue these behaviors.

The severity and impact of OCD can vary greatly among individuals. Some may experience only mild symptoms that are manageable, while others may find their daily routines severely disrupted. It's important to note that OCD can occur alongside other mental health conditions, such as depression or anxiety disorders, complicating diagnosis and treatment. Recognizing the symptoms and understanding the disorder is the first step toward seeking effective strategies for overcoming OCD.

Awareness of OCD and its symptoms is essential for those who are struggling with the disorder or who are concerned about their mental health. By understanding what OCD entails, individuals can better communicate their experiences to healthcare professionals, allowing for a more accurate diagnosis and tailored treatment plan. This knowledge serves as a foundation for implementing strategies to manage and eventually overcome OCD, fostering a path toward peace and improved mental well-being.

Types of OCD

Obsessive-Compulsive Disorder (OCD) is a complex mental health condition characterized by intrusive thoughts, images, or urges (obsessions) and repetitive behaviors or mental acts (compulsions) that individuals feel driven to perform. Understanding the various types of OCD can help individuals identify their experiences and find effective strategies for managing their symptoms. While OCD can manifest in numerous ways, there are several common categories that encapsulate the different forms it can take.

One prevalent type of OCD is contamination OCD, where individuals have an intense fear of germs, dirt, or illness. This fear can lead to excessive handwashing, avoiding certain places or people, and engaging in rituals to prevent perceived contamination. People with this type of OCD may spend significant amounts of time cleaning their surroundings, often feeling that their safety depends on these compulsive behaviors. Recognizing this pattern is crucial for individuals seeking to overcome OCD, as it allows them to challenge the irrational fears associated with cleanliness and health.

Another common form is symmetry and order OCD, characterized by an overwhelming need for things to be arranged in a particular order or symmetry. Individuals may feel discomfort or anxiety if items are not aligned or organized according to their specific preferences. This type of OCD can lead to time-consuming rituals, such as rearranging objects or counting items to achieve a sense of balance. Understanding the compulsive nature of these behaviors can aid individuals in developing strategies to confront their need for order and find peace in chaos.

Hoarding OCD is another significant subtype, where individuals struggle with the accumulation of items and a persistent inability to discard possessions. This behavior often stems from emotional attachments to objects or fears of needing them in the future. Hoarding can severely impact living conditions and relationships, leading to distress and isolation. Recognizing hoarding behaviors as a manifestation of OCD can enable individuals to seek appropriate treatment, focusing on the underlying anxieties that drive their compulsions.

Lastly, there is the type known as intrusive thoughts OCD, where individuals experience unwanted thoughts that are often violent, sexual, or blasphemous in nature. These intrusive thoughts can be distressing and lead to significant anxiety, as individuals may fear that having such thoughts reflects their character or intentions.

Understanding that these thoughts are a symptom of OCD rather than a reflection of reality is essential for individuals working to overcome this type of OCD. Strategies such as cognitive-behavioral therapy can be particularly effective in addressing and reframing these intrusive thoughts.

By recognizing the diverse types of OCD, individuals can better understand their own experiences and the specific challenges they face. This awareness is a fundamental step towards effective management and overcoming the disorder. Tailoring treatment strategies to the specific type of OCD can significantly enhance the journey toward finding peace and reclaiming control over one's life.

The Science Behind OCD

Obsessive-Compulsive Disorder (OCD) is a complex mental health condition characterized by persistent, unwanted thoughts (obsessions) and repetitive behaviors or mental acts (compulsions) that individuals feel driven to perform. The science behind OCD involves a combination of biological, psychological, and environmental factors. Neuroimaging studies have revealed that individuals with OCD often show abnormal activity in specific brain regions, particularly the orbitofrontal cortex, anterior cingulate cortex, and striatum. These areas are involved in decision-making, emotional regulation, and the processing of threats, suggesting that the brain may misinterpret normal thoughts and stimuli as significant threats that require immediate action.

Genetics also plays a crucial role in the development of OCD. Research indicates that the disorder can run in families, with first-degree relatives of individuals with OCD being more likely to develop the condition themselves. Several genes have been implicated in OCD, particularly those involved in serotonin regulation.

Serotonin is a neurotransmitter that plays a key role in mood and anxiety regulation. When serotonin levels are disrupted, it can lead to the heightened anxiety and compulsive behaviors characteristic of OCD. Understanding the genetic components of OCD can help in developing targeted treatments and interventions.

Environmental factors can contribute to the onset and exacerbation of OCD symptoms. Traumatic experiences, significant life changes, or chronic stress can trigger the development of OCD in individuals predisposed to the disorder. For example, research has shown that children who experience infections, particularly streptococcal infections, may develop OCD symptoms in a condition known as Pediatric Autoimmune Neuropsychiatric Disorders Associated with Streptococcal Infections (PANDAS). This highlights the importance of considering both biological and environmental interactions in the treatment and management of OCD.

Cognitive-behavioral therapy (CBT) is the most effective treatment for OCD, particularly a specific form known as Exposure and Response Prevention (ERP). This therapeutic approach works by gradually exposing individuals to their fears while preventing the corresponding compulsive behaviors.

Through this process, patients learn to tolerate the anxiety associated with their obsessions without resorting to compulsions, ultimately reducing the power of the obsessions over time. Additionally, pharmacological treatments, such as selective serotonin reuptake inhibitors (SSRIs), can help alleviate symptoms by increasing serotonin levels in the brain, providing another avenue for recovery.

Understanding the science behind OCD is essential for those seeking to overcome the disorder. By recognizing the interplay of biological, genetic, and environmental factors, individuals can better comprehend their experiences and the underlying mechanisms of their symptoms.

This knowledge empowers individuals to engage more effectively with treatment options, whether they choose therapy, medication, or a combination of both. With the right strategies and support, it is possible to manage and significantly reduce the impact of OCD on one's daily life.

How To Overcome OCD

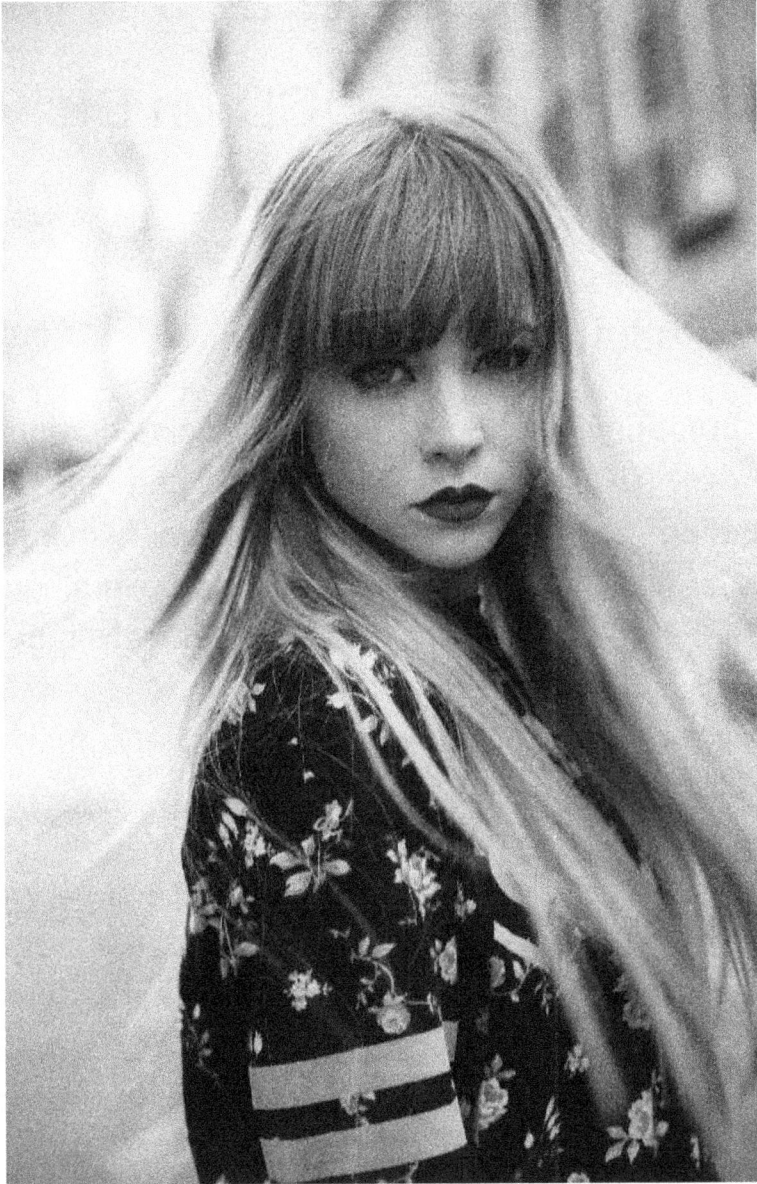

Chapter 2

The Impact of OCD on Daily Life

Emotional Effects

Emotional effects of obsessive-compulsive disorder (OCD) can be profound and pervasive, impacting not only the individual experiencing the disorder but also their relationships and overall quality of life. People with OCD often find themselves caught in a cycle of intrusive thoughts and compulsive behaviors, leading to heightened anxiety, fear, and distress.

This emotional turmoil can create a sense of isolation, as individuals may feel misunderstood by those around them, unable to articulate the depth of their internal struggles. Recognizing these emotional effects is the first step toward developing effective strategies for overcoming OCD.

One of the most significant emotional challenges faced by those with OCD is the overwhelming anxiety generated by intrusive thoughts. These thoughts can manifest in various forms, often revolving around fears of harm, contamination, or loss of control. The distress caused by these thoughts can lead to compulsive behaviors designed to mitigate perceived threats, ironically reinforcing the cycle of anxiety.

Understanding this relationship between thoughts and emotions is crucial for individuals seeking to break free from OCD's grip, as it helps in recognizing that the thoughts are not a reflection of reality but rather a product of the disorder.

Depression is another common emotional effect associated with OCD. The relentless nature of obsessive thoughts and compulsive actions can lead to feelings of hopelessness and despair. Individuals may find themselves withdrawing from activities they once enjoyed or isolating themselves from friends and family due to embarrassment or shame.

This emotional state can create a vicious cycle, where the symptoms of OCD exacerbate feelings of depression, leading to further withdrawal and avoidance. Addressing these emotional effects through therapy and support is essential for breaking this cycle and fostering a sense of connection and fulfillment.

The impact of OCD on interpersonal relationships cannot be overstated. Loved ones may struggle to understand the complexities of the disorder, leading to frustration and tension. Individuals with OCD may feel guilty for the burden their condition places on others, which can further deepen feelings of shame and isolation.

Effective communication and education about OCD are critical in fostering understanding and support within relationships. Encouraging open dialogues about the emotional challenges associated with OCD can help bridge gaps in understanding, ultimately strengthening bonds and promoting a supportive environment for recovery.

In coping with the emotional effects of OCD, developing healthy coping strategies is vital. Mindfulness practices, cognitive-behavioral therapy, and exposure and response prevention are some approaches that can help individuals manage their emotions effectively. These strategies empower individuals to confront their fears without resorting to compulsive behaviors, gradually reducing anxiety and emotional distress.

Additionally, building a strong support system of friends, family, or support groups can provide individuals with the necessary encouragement and understanding as they navigate their journey toward overcoming OCD. By addressing the emotional effects head-on, individuals can pave the way for healing and reclaiming their lives.

Social Consequences

Social consequences of Obsessive-Compulsive Disorder (OCD) can profoundly impact an individual's daily life. People with OCD often find themselves trapped in a cycle of compulsions and obsessions, which can lead to withdrawal from social situations, strained relationships, and feelings of isolation.

Understanding these social ramifications is crucial for both individuals struggling with OCD and their loved ones, as it can foster empathy and encourage strategies to mitigate these challenges.

One of the most significant social consequences is the tendency for individuals with OCD to avoid situations that trigger their obsessions. This avoidance behavior can lead to missed opportunities for social interaction, making it difficult to maintain friendships or engage in community activities.

Over time, this withdrawal can create a sense of loneliness and alienation, reinforcing the disorder's grip on the individual. The social fabric of a person's life becomes frayed, as they may feel incapable of participating in events that others take for granted.

Relationships can also suffer due to the misunderstandings surrounding OCD. Friends and family may struggle to comprehend the nature of the disorder, sometimes interpreting compulsive behaviors as mere quirks or stubbornness. This lack of understanding can lead to frustration and resentment on both sides.

Loved ones may feel helpless, while the person with OCD might feel judged or unsupported. Open communication about the disorder is essential for fostering understanding and compassion, which can help mitigate the strain on these important relationships.

The stigma associated with mental health disorders, including OCD, can exacerbate these social consequences. Individuals may fear being labeled or judged, leading them to hide their symptoms rather than seeking help. This secrecy not only increases feelings of shame but also prevents individuals from accessing support networks that could aid in their recovery.

Addressing the stigma surrounding OCD is vital for encouraging individuals to share their experiences and seek the assistance they need, creating a more supportive environment for healing.

Lastly, engaging in therapy or support groups can provide a remedy for the social consequences of OCD. These settings allow individuals to connect with others who share similar experiences, fostering a sense of community and understanding.

Therapy can also equip individuals with coping strategies to help manage their symptoms in social situations, reducing avoidance behaviors. By actively participating in these supportive environments, individuals can rebuild their social connections and work towards overcoming the isolating effects of OCD, ultimately leading to a more fulfilling life.

Occupational Challenges

Occupational challenges for individuals with obsessive-compulsive disorder (OCD) can significantly impact their professional lives. Many people with OCD experience intrusive thoughts and compulsive behaviors that can interfere with their ability to focus, complete tasks, or collaborate with colleagues. The workplace environment often adds additional stressors, making it essential for individuals to develop effective strategies to manage their symptoms while maintaining productivity. Understanding the specific occupational challenges faced by those with OCD is vital for creating a supportive work environment.

One significant challenge is the demand for high levels of concentration and attention to detail. Many jobs require individuals to perform repetitive tasks or meet strict deadlines. For someone with OCD, the need for perfection and fear of making mistakes can lead to excessive time spent on tasks, rechecking work, or engaging in compulsive behaviors that disrupt workflow. This can result in lower productivity and increased anxiety, further exacerbating the symptoms of OCD. Identifying these challenges early on can help individuals develop coping mechanisms that allow them to navigate their work responsibilities more efficiently.

Social interactions in the workplace can also present difficulties for those with OCD. Anxiety surrounding social situations may lead to avoidance behaviors, making it hard to engage with colleagues or participate in team activities. The fear of judgment or misunderstanding can exacerbate feelings of loneliness and isolation. Building relationships with coworkers is crucial for professional growth, so finding ways to ease social anxiety, such as practicing mindfulness or role-playing scenarios, can help create a more comfortable atmosphere for individuals with OCD.

Time management is another area where occupational challenges often arise. The compulsive need to perform certain rituals can consume significant amounts of time, leaving little room for completing essential job functions. Individuals may struggle to balance their workload due to the time lost to compulsions.

Implementing structured schedules and breaking tasks into manageable segments can provide a sense of control and help reduce the overwhelming nature of work responsibilities. Additionally, using organizational tools can keep individuals on track and minimize distractions.

Lastly, it is essential for employers and colleagues to foster a supportive work environment for those with OCD. Encouraging open communication about mental health can help reduce stigma and promote understanding among team members. Providing accommodations, such as flexible work hours or the option to work in quieter spaces, can also assist individuals in managing their symptoms more effectively.

By creating a culture of empathy and support, workplaces can empower individuals with OCD to overcome their occupational challenges, ultimately leading to improved job satisfaction and overall well-being.

How To Overcome OCD

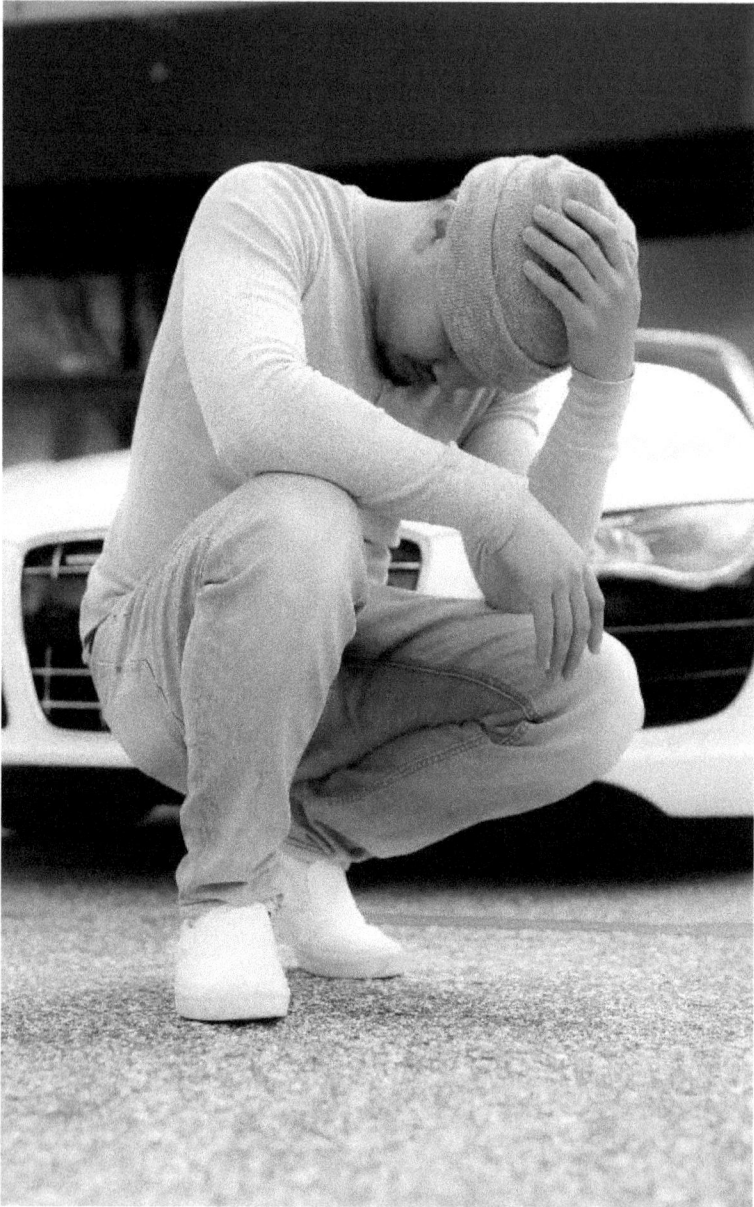

Chapter 3
Recognizing Triggers

Common Triggers

Understanding the common triggers of Obsessive-Compulsive Disorder (OCD) is essential for those seeking to manage their symptoms effectively. Triggers can vary significantly from one individual to another, but they typically involve situations, thoughts, or environments that provoke obsessive thoughts and compulsive behaviors. By recognizing these triggers, individuals can develop strategies to confront and cope with their OCD, leading to a more peaceful existence.

One prevalent trigger for many people with OCD is stress. High-pressure situations, whether at work, in personal relationships, or related to life transitions, can exacerbate obsessive thoughts and compulsive rituals. Stress can lead to increased anxiety, which may drive individuals to engage in their compulsions as a way to alleviate discomfort.

Identifying stressors in daily life is crucial, as it allows individuals to create a plan for managing stress through relaxation techniques, time management, or seeking support from friends and family.

Another common trigger is specific environments or locations. Certain places may evoke memories or feelings associated with past obsessions, prompting a surge of anxiety. For example, an individual may find that entering a public restroom triggers intrusive thoughts about contamination, leading to compulsive handwashing or avoidance of the situation altogether.

Learning to recognize these environments and gradually facing them in a controlled manner can be a key part of exposure therapy, a common treatment for OCD that encourages individuals to confront their fears.

Intrusive thoughts themselves can also serve as powerful triggers. These thoughts are often unwanted and distressing, leading the individual to engage in compulsive behaviors to neutralize the anxiety they cause.

For instance, someone may experience a sudden, irrational fear of harming a loved one, prompting them to seek reassurance or engage in rituals to prevent this from happening. Understanding that these thoughts are a symptom of OCD and not a reflection of personal values is crucial in reducing their power and influence.

Lastly, personal relationships can act as triggers for those with OCD. Interactions with loved ones may become strained as compulsions interfere with daily life. For instance, a partner may feel overwhelmed by the repetitive questions or rituals of someone with OCD, which can lead to frustration and misunderstandings.

Open communication about OCD and its effects can help diminish these triggers, allowing for a supportive environment where both parties can navigate the challenges together. Building a strong support network is vital for individuals with OCD as it provides both understanding and encouragement in their journey toward recovery.

Personal Trigger Identification

Personal Trigger Identification is a crucial step in managing Obsessive-Compulsive Disorder (OCD) and finding effective strategies to cope with its symptoms. Triggers are specific situations, thoughts, or stimuli that provoke obsessive thoughts and compulsive behaviors.

By identifying these triggers, individuals can better understand their OCD patterns and develop tailored coping mechanisms. The process begins with self-reflection, where individuals must pay close attention to their thoughts and feelings during daily activities.

Keeping a journal can be particularly helpful, as it allows for the documentation of situations that lead to heightened anxiety and compulsive responses.

Once individuals have begun to document their experiences, the next step is to categorize their triggers. Triggers can be grouped into various categories, such as environmental, social, emotional, or cognitive.

Environmental triggers may include clutter, specific locations, or even certain sounds, while social triggers might involve interactions with specific people or situations. Emotional triggers often relate to feelings of stress, sadness, or fear, while cognitive triggers are related to intrusive thoughts. By understanding the categories of their triggers, individuals can pinpoint patterns that contribute to their OCD symptoms.

After categorizing triggers, it is essential to evaluate their intensity and frequency. Some triggers may lead to mild discomfort, while others can cause significant distress and compulsive behaviors. This evaluation process helps individuals prioritize which triggers to address first.

By focusing on the most impactful triggers, individuals can create a more manageable approach to their OCD treatment. Additionally, understanding the intensity of triggers can inform the development of coping strategies, allowing individuals to gradually expose themselves to these triggers in a controlled manner.

Developing coping strategies to manage identified triggers is a vital part of the personal trigger identification process. Exposure and Response Prevention (ERP) therapy is one commonly recommended approach. This method involves gradually exposing oneself to a trigger while resisting the urge to engage in compulsive behaviors. By practicing this technique in a supportive environment, individuals can reduce their anxiety over time. Other strategies may include mindfulness exercises, deep breathing techniques, or cognitive restructuring to challenge negative thoughts associated with triggers.

Finally, personal trigger identification is an ongoing process that requires patience and adaptability. As individuals progress in their journey to manage OCD, new triggers may emerge, or existing ones may become less prominent. Regularly revisiting and updating the list of triggers is essential to ensure that coping strategies remain effective. Support from mental health professionals, as well as participation in support groups, can also provide valuable insights and encouragement. By actively engaging in personal trigger identification, individuals can take significant steps toward overcoming OCD and achieving a greater sense of peace in their lives.

Avoidance vs. Confrontation

Avoidance and confrontation are two distinct strategies individuals often employ when dealing with obsessive-compulsive disorder (OCD). Understanding the differences between these approaches is crucial for effective management of OCD symptoms. Avoidance involves steering clear of situations, thoughts, or objects that trigger anxiety or compulsive behaviors.

This strategy may provide short-term relief, but it often reinforces the cycle of OCD, making the condition more entrenched. On the other hand, confrontation entails facing these triggers directly, which can be uncomfortable but is necessary for long-term recovery.

When individuals with OCD choose avoidance, they may believe they are protecting themselves from distress. For example, someone with a fear of contamination might avoid public places or refuse to touch certain objects. This behavior may temporarily reduce anxiety, but it also limits their daily life and reinforces the belief that these triggers are dangerous.

As a result, the individual may become increasingly restricted in their activities, leading to social isolation and a decrease in overall quality of life. Consequently, avoidance can create a false sense of safety that ultimately exacerbates OCD symptoms.

In contrast, confrontation requires a willingness to face fears head-on. This approach often involves exposure therapy, a common and effective treatment for OCD. Exposure therapy encourages individuals to gradually engage with their fears in a controlled and supportive environment. For instance, someone with a fear of germs might start by touching a mildly contaminated object and then gradually progress to more challenging situations. While this process can initially increase anxiety, consistent confrontation helps to desensitize the individual to their fears, ultimately reducing the intensity of their OCD symptoms over time.

Confrontation also plays a critical role in cognitive restructuring, a technique used to challenge and change irrational beliefs associated with OCD. By confronting the thoughts that fuel compulsive behaviors, individuals can learn to reframe their thinking and develop healthier coping mechanisms.

Over time, this approach fosters resilience and empowers individuals to regain control over their lives, rather than allowing OCD to dictate their actions. The journey of confrontation may be daunting, but it is a vital step toward achieving lasting peace.

Ultimately, the choice between avoidance and confrontation is one that individuals with OCD must navigate carefully. While avoidance may seem like the easier path, it often leads to greater entrapment in the disorder. Embracing confrontation, though challenging, is essential for breaking the cycle of compulsions and obsessions. By understanding the value of facing fears and seeking help through therapeutic techniques, individuals can embark on a journey toward recovery, equipped with the tools to find lasting peace and fulfillment in their lives.

How To Overcome OCD

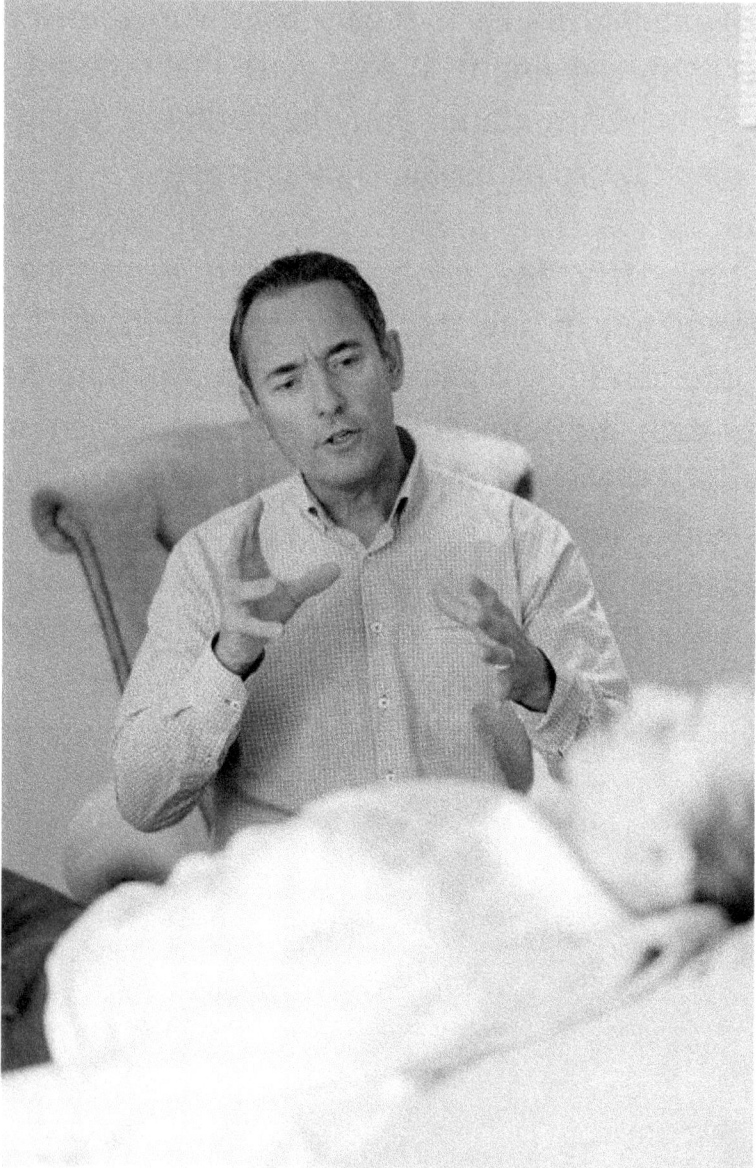

Chapter 4

Seeking Professional Help

Types of Therapies

Cognitive Behavioral Therapy (CBT) is one of the most widely recognized and effective treatments for Obsessive-Compulsive Disorder (OCD). This therapy focuses on changing the negative thought patterns and behaviors that contribute to OCD symptoms. Through CBT, individuals learn to identify their obsessions and compulsions, which allows them to challenge and reframe these thoughts.

Techniques such as exposure and response prevention (ERP) are integral to this approach, helping individuals gradually face their fears while refraining from engaging in compulsive behaviors. This method has shown significant success in reducing the intensity of OCD symptoms and empowering individuals to regain control over their lives.

Another effective therapy for OCD is Acceptance and Commitment Therapy (ACT). ACT encourages individuals to accept their thoughts and feelings rather than fight against them. This therapy emphasizes mindfulness and the importance of living in accordance with personal values, despite the presence of distressing thoughts.

By fostering psychological flexibility, ACT helps individuals develop a healthier relationship with their obsessions, allowing them to take committed action toward their goals without being hindered by their OCD. This approach can be particularly beneficial for those who struggle with the shame and guilt often associated with OCD, as it promotes self-compassion and acceptance.

Mindfulness-based therapies are gaining traction as effective options for managing OCD symptoms. These approaches integrate mindfulness practices with traditional therapeutic techniques to help individuals cultivate present-moment awareness and reduce anxiety. Mindfulness encourages individuals to observe their thoughts without judgment, which can diminish the power of obsessions and compulsions.

By practicing mindfulness, individuals can learn to detach from their anxious thoughts and reduce the urgency to perform compulsive behaviors. This practice can lead to a greater sense of calm and a more balanced emotional state, making it easier to cope with OCD.

In addition to these therapies, medication can also play a crucial role in the treatment of OCD. Selective serotonin reuptake inhibitors (SSRIs) are commonly prescribed to help regulate serotonin levels in the brain, which can alleviate obsessive thoughts and compulsive behaviors. While medication is not a standalone solution, it can be an effective adjunct to therapy, particularly when symptoms are severe. It is essential for individuals to work closely with their healthcare providers to find the right medication and dosage, as responses to medication can vary widely among individuals.

Finally, support groups and peer-led interventions can provide additional layers of support for those dealing with OCD. These groups create a safe space for individuals to share their experiences, challenges, and coping strategies.

Connecting with others who understand the unique struggles of living with OCD can foster a sense of community and reduce feelings of isolation. Through shared stories and encouragement, participants can gain new insights into their own experiences and learn from the successes of others. Support groups can be a valuable complement to formal therapy, reinforcing the idea that individuals are not alone in their journey toward overcoming OCD.

Medication Options

For individuals grappling with Obsessive-Compulsive Disorder (OCD), medication can play a crucial role in managing symptoms and improving overall quality of life. The most commonly prescribed medications for OCD belong to a class called selective serotonin reuptake inhibitors (SSRIs). These medications work by increasing the levels of serotonin in the brain, a neurotransmitter that is often imbalanced in those with OCD. Some of the most frequently prescribed SSRIs for OCD include fluoxetine, fluvoxamine, and sertraline. It is essential for individuals to consult with a healthcare professional to determine the most appropriate medication based on their specific symptoms and medical history.

In addition to SSRIs, another class of medications known as clomipramine, a tricyclic antidepressant, has also shown effectiveness in treating OCD. Clomipramine has been found to reduce obsessive thoughts and compulsive behaviors in many patients. While it can be effective, it may also come with a higher risk of side effects compared to SSRIs.

Therefore, it's important for individuals to weigh the benefits and potential drawbacks of each medication with their healthcare provider. Understanding the unique properties of these medications can empower individuals to make informed decisions about their treatment options.

Before starting any medication, it is crucial to have thorough discussions with a healthcare professional about potential side effects, interactions with other medications, and the length of time it may take for the medication to show effects. Many individuals may need to try different medications or dosages to find the right fit for their needs.

This process can require patience, as it often takes several weeks for the full benefits of the medication to be realized. Monitoring and adjusting the treatment plan with the guidance of a healthcare provider can significantly enhance the chances of finding an effective medication regimen.

It is also important to note that medication is often most effective when combined with therapy, particularly cognitive-behavioral therapy (CBT), which is a well-established treatment for OCD. The combination of medication and therapy can address both the biological and psychological aspects of the disorder, leading to more comprehensive symptom relief.

Individuals are encouraged to explore this combined approach, as it may lead to improved outcomes and a greater sense of control over their OCD symptoms.

Lastly, individuals should remain open to reviewing their treatment options regularly. As symptoms evolve or as life circumstances change, the effectiveness of a medication may also shift.

Maintaining ongoing communication with healthcare providers and being proactive about treatment adjustments can be key to long-term management of OCD. By understanding the various medication options and their potential impacts, individuals can take significant steps towards reclaiming their lives from the grasp of OCD.

Finding the Right Therapist

Finding the right therapist is a crucial step in overcoming Obsessive-Compulsive Disorder (OCD). The therapeutic relationship can significantly impact the effectiveness of treatment, and choosing someone who understands your specific needs and experiences is essential.

When searching for a therapist, consider their qualifications, experience, and therapeutic approach. Look for professionals who specialize in OCD and are familiar with evidence-based treatments such as Cognitive Behavioral Therapy (CBT) and Exposure and Response Prevention (ERP).

One of the first steps in your search should be to gather recommendations. Speak with your primary care physician, friends, or family members who may have experience with mental health professionals. Online directories and mental health organizations can also provide valuable resources. When you compile a list of potential therapists, take the time to research their backgrounds, including education, training, and areas of specialization. Understanding their approach to treating OCD will help you make an informed decision.

During the initial consultation, assess not only the therapist's qualifications but also your comfort level with them. A good therapeutic alliance is built on trust and open communication. Pay attention to how the therapist listens to your concerns and whether they validate your experiences. It is important that you feel safe discussing your thoughts and feelings without fear of judgment. If the therapist makes you feel uneasy or dismissive, it may be a sign to continue your search.

Consider the logistical aspects of therapy as well. Inquire about the therapist's availability, session frequency, and whether they accept your insurance. Accessibility can play a significant role in your commitment to treatment. Furthermore, think about whether you prefer in-person sessions or if teletherapy options are more suitable for your lifestyle. The convenience of scheduling and location can affect your overall experience and engagement in the therapeutic process.

Finally, remember that finding the right therapist can take time. It is not uncommon to meet with multiple professionals before discovering the one who fits your needs. Be patient with yourself throughout this journey. Each therapist brings a unique perspective and approach, and your experiences will guide you toward a practitioner who resonates with you. Prioritizing the right therapeutic fit is an essential part of your journey to overcoming OCD and finding peace.

How To Overcome OCD

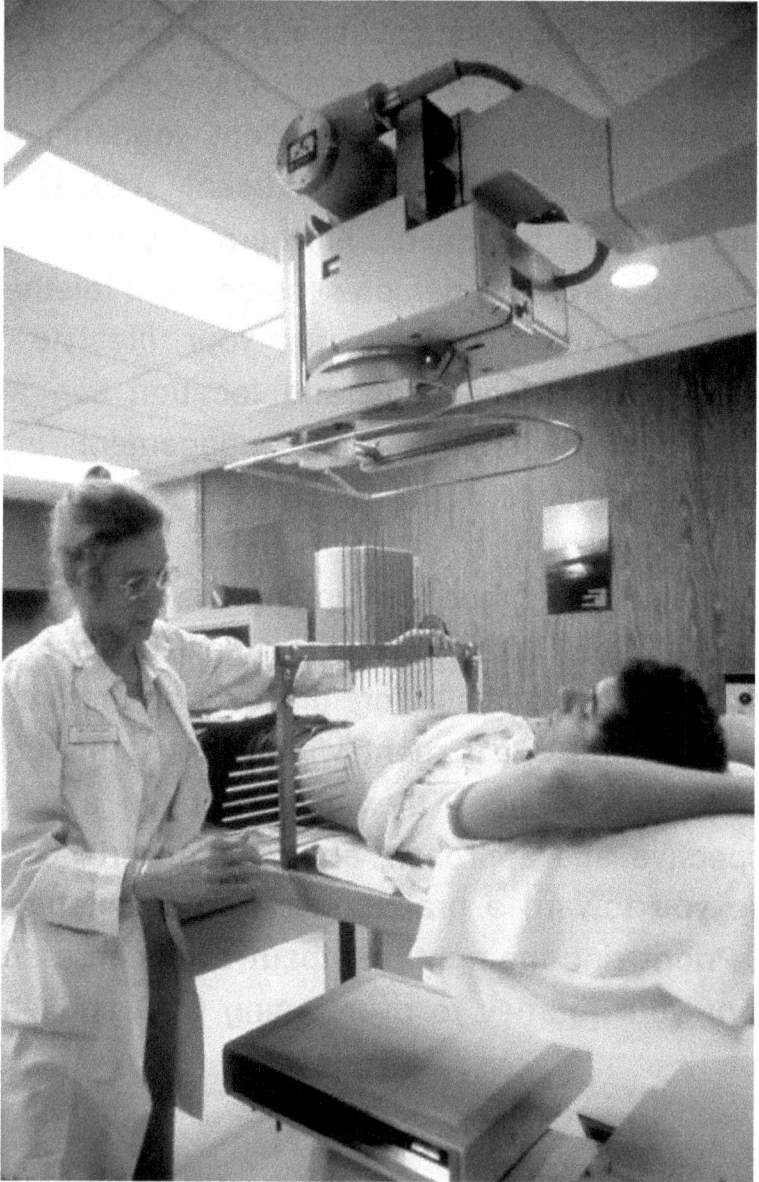

Chapter 5

Cognitive Behavioral Therapy (CBT)

Principles of CBT

Cognitive Behavioral Therapy (CBT) is a structured, time-limited psychotherapeutic approach that has proven effective in treating various mental health conditions, including Obsessive-Compulsive Disorder (OCD). The core principle of CBT revolves around the understanding that our thoughts, emotions, and behaviors are interlinked.

When individuals experience OCD, they often face intrusive thoughts that lead to anxiety and compulsive behaviors aimed at alleviating that anxiety. CBT helps individuals recognize the cognitive distortions fueling their obsessions and teaches them to challenge and modify these thoughts.

Central to CBT is the concept of cognitive restructuring. This involves identifying negative thought patterns and replacing them with more balanced and realistic thoughts. For individuals with OCD, this process can help dismantle the irrational beliefs that often accompany their obsessions. By systematically examining these thoughts and their validity, clients can learn to reduce the power these thoughts hold over them. This shift not only alleviates anxiety but also diminishes the compulsive behaviors that often follow obsessive thoughts.

Another fundamental aspect of CBT is exposure and response prevention (ERP). This technique involves gradually exposing individuals to the situations or thoughts that trigger their OCD while preventing the accompanying compulsive behaviors. The goal of ERP is to help individuals learn that their fears are unfounded and that they can tolerate the anxiety without resorting to compulsions. Over time, this exposure leads to a decrease in anxiety levels and an increase in the individual's sense of control over their thoughts and behaviors.

CBT also emphasizes the importance of self-monitoring and homework assignments. Clients are encouraged to keep a record of their thoughts, feelings, and behaviors, which can provide valuable insights into their patterns of OCD. Through these assignments, individuals can practice the skills they learn in therapy and apply them to real-life situations. This active engagement in the therapeutic process enhances the effectiveness of CBT, as it allows clients to reinforce the strategies they have learned and track their progress over time.

Lastly, the collaborative nature of the therapeutic relationship in CBT is essential. Therapists work closely with clients to establish goals and develop personalized strategies that align with the individual's unique experiences with OCD. This partnership fosters a sense of accountability and support, which can be crucial for clients as they navigate the challenges of overcoming their OCD. By grounding the therapy in collaboration and mutual understanding, CBT empowers individuals to take an active role in their recovery journey, ultimately leading to lasting change and improved well-being.

Exposure and Response Prevention (ERP)

Exposure and Response Prevention (ERP) is a cornerstone therapeutic approach for individuals struggling with Obsessive-Compulsive Disorder (OCD). This method is rooted in cognitive-behavioral therapy and focuses on gradually exposing individuals to the sources of their anxiety while preventing the compulsive behaviors that they typically engage in to alleviate that anxiety.

The primary goal of ERP is to help individuals confront their fears in a structured and supportive environment, ultimately leading to a reduction in anxiety and the compulsions associated with it.

The exposure component of ERP involves carefully planned and systematic encounters with the obsessions that trigger anxiety. This can range from confronting specific fears to engaging with situations that provoke obsessive thoughts.

The process begins with identifying these fears and developing a hierarchy of exposure tasks, starting with less anxiety-provoking scenarios and gradually moving toward more challenging situations. This gradual exposure allows individuals to build confidence and resilience as they face their fears in a controlled manner.

In conjunction with exposure, response prevention is a critical aspect of ERP. It involves refraining from engaging in compulsive behaviors that serve as temporary relief from anxiety. For instance, if an individual feels compelled to wash their hands repeatedly due to fears of contamination, ERP will encourage them to resist this compulsion while remaining in the anxiety-provoking situation. Over time, this practice helps individuals learn that their anxiety will diminish without the need for compulsive actions, breaking the cycle of OCD.

ERP is most effective when implemented under the guidance of a trained mental health professional who can provide support and encouragement throughout the process. Therapists work closely with individuals to ensure that exposures are manageable and tailored to their specific triggers.

Additionally, they help individuals develop coping strategies to manage the discomfort that arises during exposure sessions. This supportive relationship can enhance the effectiveness of ERP and provide individuals with the tools they need to face their fears.

While ERP can be challenging and may initially increase anxiety levels, research has consistently shown it to be one of the most effective treatments for OCD. As individuals progress through their treatment, they often experience a significant decrease in their symptoms and an increased sense of control over their lives. By committing to the principles of exposure and response prevention, individuals can take meaningful steps toward overcoming OCD and finding the peace they seek.

Self-Help CBT Techniques

Self-Help Cognitive Behavioral Therapy (CBT) techniques are valuable tools for individuals grappling with Obsessive-Compulsive Disorder (OCD). These techniques empower sufferers to take control of their thoughts and behaviors, fostering a sense of autonomy and self-efficacy.

By integrating these methods into daily life, individuals can significantly reduce the impact of OCD symptoms and work towards achieving a more peaceful state of mind.

One of the foundational strategies in self-help CBT is exposure and response prevention (ERP). This technique involves gradually exposing oneself to the thoughts, images, and situations that trigger OCD symptoms, while simultaneously refraining from engaging in compulsive behaviors.

For example, if an individual has an obsession with cleanliness, they might start by touching a surface they perceive as dirty and then resist the urge to wash their hands immediately. This process helps to diminish the anxiety associated with the obsessive thoughts over time, strengthening the individual's ability to manage their OCD symptoms.

Another effective technique is cognitive restructuring, which focuses on identifying and challenging irrational beliefs related to OCD.

Individuals can learn to recognize distorted thinking patterns, such as catastrophizing or all-or-nothing thinking, and replace them with more balanced and realistic thoughts.

Individuals can learn to recognize distorted thinking patterns, such as catastrophizing or all-or-nothing thinking, and replace them with more balanced and realistic thoughts.

For instance, instead of thinking, "If I don't check the locks ten times, my house will be broken into," one could reframe this to, "I have checked the locks, and my home is secure." This shift in perspective helps to reduce the power of obsessive thoughts and lessens the need for compulsive behaviors.

Mindfulness practices also play a crucial role in self-help CBT for OCD. By cultivating an awareness of the present moment and accepting thoughts without judgment, individuals can create distance from their obsessions. Techniques such as deep breathing, meditation, and body scans can help ground individuals when they feel overwhelmed by intrusive thoughts.

Mindfulness encourages a compassionate attitude towards oneself, fostering resilience against the negative self-talk that often accompanies OCD.

Lastly, journaling can serve as a powerful self-help tool for those with OCD. Keeping a daily log of thoughts, feelings, and compulsions allows individuals to track their progress and identify patterns in their OCD. Writing can also provide a safe outlet for expressing fears and anxieties, which can help to reduce their intensity. By reflecting on their experiences, individuals can gain insight into their triggers and develop more effective coping strategies, thus further enhancing their journey towards overcoming OCD.

How To Overcome OCD

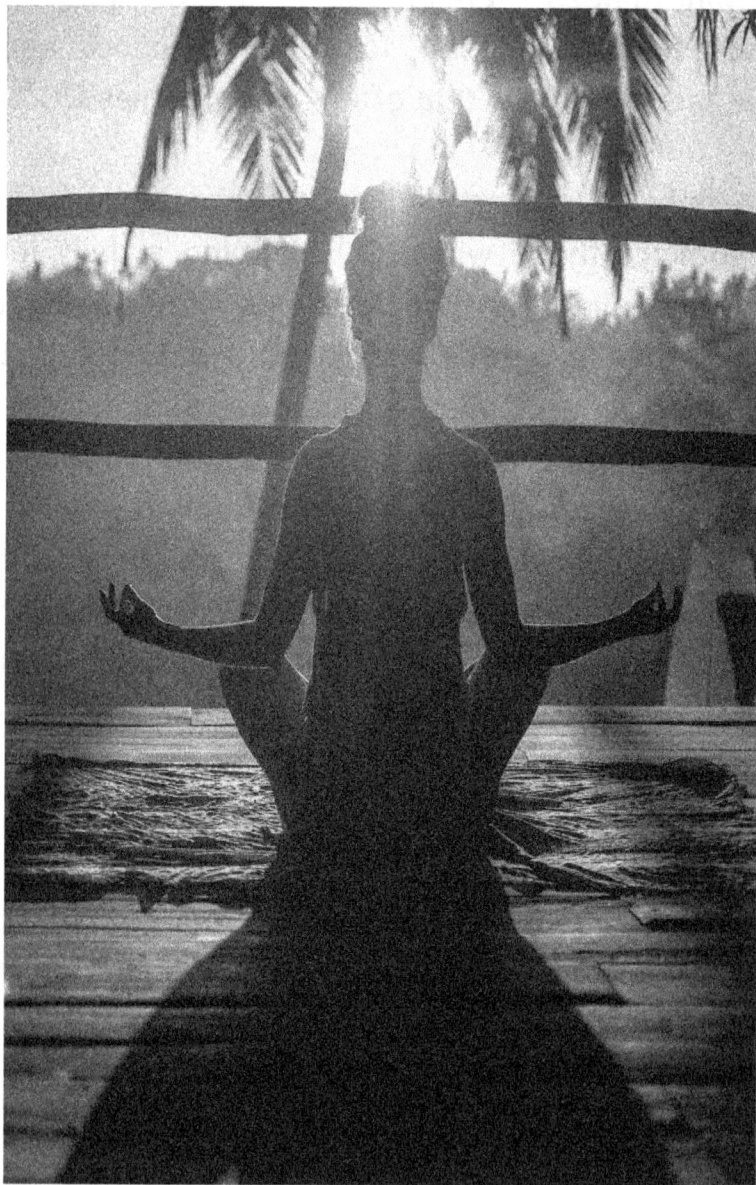

Chapter 6

Mindfulness and Relaxation Techniques

Importance of Mindfulness

Mindfulness is a practice rooted in ancient traditions that has gained significant attention in modern psychology, particularly in its application to overcoming anxiety disorders such as Obsessive-Compulsive Disorder (OCD). It involves maintaining a moment-by-moment awareness of our thoughts, feelings, and surroundings without judgment.

For those struggling with OCD, mindfulness can serve as a powerful tool to break the cycle of obsessive thinking and compulsive behaviors. By fostering an attitude of acceptance rather than resistance, individuals can learn to observe their thoughts and emotions without becoming overwhelmed by them.

One of the key benefits of mindfulness is its ability to enhance emotional regulation. People with OCD often experience intense emotions, such as fear or anxiety, triggered by their obsessions. Mindfulness encourages individuals to acknowledge these emotions without automatically reacting to them. This practice allows for a pause between the thought and the response, creating space to choose healthier coping strategies. By recognizing that thoughts are not facts, individuals can reduce the power that their obsessions hold over them.

Mindfulness also promotes self-compassion, which is crucial for those dealing with OCD. Individuals often feel shame or guilt about their intrusive thoughts and compulsive behaviors. Mindfulness encourages a non-judgmental attitude toward oneself, fostering kindness and understanding. This shift in perspective can help individuals recognize that they are not alone in their struggles and that experiencing unwanted thoughts does not define their character. By cultivating self-compassion through mindfulness, individuals can alleviate some of the stigma they place on themselves, making it easier to confront their OCD.

Incorporating mindfulness into daily routines can be straightforward yet transformative. Simple practices such as mindful breathing, body scans, or mindful walking can be integrated into everyday life. These exercises can help ground individuals in the present moment, making it easier to detach from obsessive thoughts and the compulsion to act on them. Consistent practice can enhance the effectiveness of other therapeutic strategies, such as cognitive-behavioral therapy, by reinforcing the skills learned in treatment and providing additional tools to manage anxiety.

Ultimately, the importance of mindfulness in overcoming OCD lies in its ability to empower individuals. By developing a mindful approach, individuals can gain a greater sense of control over their thoughts and behaviors. This empowerment fosters resilience, enabling them to face challenges with a clearer mind and a more compassionate heart. As they learn to navigate their OCD with mindfulness, they can move closer to finding peace and reclaiming their lives from the grips of the disorder.

Breathing Exercises

Breathing exercises are a powerful tool for managing the symptoms of obsessive-compulsive disorder (OCD). They can serve as an effective method to reduce anxiety and bring about a sense of calm when intrusive thoughts arise. By focusing on the breath, individuals can anchor themselves in the present moment, which is crucial for combating the overwhelming feelings that OCD often brings. These exercises can be practiced anywhere and at any time, making them a convenient option for those seeking relief from their symptoms.

One of the simplest breathing techniques is diaphragmatic breathing, also known as abdominal or deep breathing. To practice this, find a comfortable position, either seated or lying down. Place one hand on your chest and the other on your abdomen. Inhale deeply through your nose, allowing your abdomen to rise while keeping your chest relatively still. Exhale slowly through your mouth, feeling your abdomen fall. This technique encourages full oxygen exchange, which can help lower heart rate and blood pressure, ultimately reducing feelings of anxiety.

Another effective method is the 4-7-8 breathing technique, which promotes relaxation and helps to quiet the mind. Begin by inhaling through your nose for a count of four, then hold your breath for a count of seven. Finally, exhale slowly through your mouth for a count of eight. This cycle can be repeated several times. The rhythmic pattern of inhaling and exhaling can create a meditative state, allowing individuals to detach from their obsessive thoughts and focus on their breath instead.

Incorporating breathing exercises into daily routines can also enhance their effectiveness. Setting aside specific times each day to practice these techniques can help establish a sense of control over one's symptoms.

Additionally, pairing breathing exercises with mindfulness or grounding techniques can further enhance their impact. For instance, after completing a breathing exercise, individuals might take a moment to notice their surroundings, engaging their senses to draw their attention away from distressing thoughts.

Ultimately, mastering breathing exercises takes practice and patience. It is essential for individuals to find the techniques that resonate with them and to remain committed to incorporating them into their life. Over time, these exercises can become a reliable coping mechanism, enabling individuals with OCD to navigate their anxieties more effectively. By cultivating a regular practice of breathing exercises, individuals can work towards achieving a greater sense of peace and control over their OCD symptoms.

Guided Imagery

Guided imagery is a therapeutic technique that utilizes visualization to promote relaxation and mental clarity. It involves creating mental images that evoke a sense of peace and tranquility, helping individuals to manage anxiety and obsessive thoughts often associated with Obsessive-Compulsive Disorder (OCD). By engaging in guided imagery, individuals can learn to redirect their focus from distressing thoughts to calming scenarios, ultimately reducing the impact of OCD symptoms.

The process of guided imagery typically begins with finding a quiet and comfortable space. Participants are encouraged to close their eyes and take a few deep breaths, allowing their bodies to relax. A trained therapist or a recorded session may then guide them through a series of visualizations. These may include imagining a serene landscape, such as a beach or a peaceful forest, where they can escape from their intrusive thoughts. The vividness of these images can help create a strong emotional response, leading to a greater sense of calm.

Incorporating guided imagery into a daily routine can significantly enhance its effectiveness. Practicing this technique regularly allows individuals to build a mental library of calming images they can draw upon whenever they feel overwhelmed. As they become more adept at evoking these peaceful scenarios, they may find that their ability to cope with OCD symptoms improves. This practice not only aids in managing anxiety but also contributes to a greater sense of control over one's thoughts and reactions.

Research has shown that guided imagery can be particularly effective when combined with other therapeutic approaches, such as cognitive-behavioral therapy (CBT). While CBT addresses the cognitive distortions associated with OCD, guided imagery can serve as a complementary tool to help individuals relax and process their feelings. By integrating these methods, individuals may experience a more comprehensive approach to overcoming their OCD, leading to sustained improvements in their mental health.

Overall, guided imagery is a valuable technique for those seeking to manage OCD. It empowers individuals to create their own mental sanctuary, providing them with a tool to combat anxiety and obsessive thoughts. By regularly practicing guided imagery, individuals can foster a greater sense of peace and resilience, making significant strides in their journey toward overcoming the challenges posed by OCD.

How To Overcome OCD

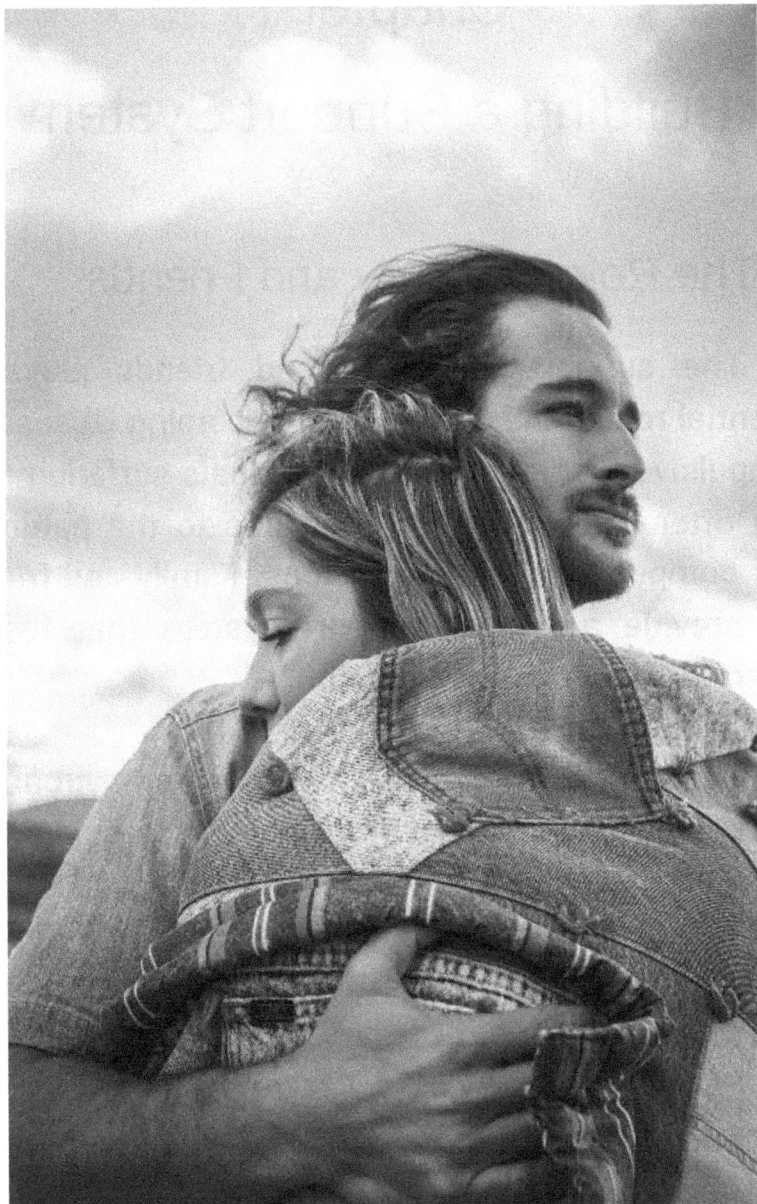

Chapter 7

Building a Support System

The Role of Family and Friends

The support of family and friends plays an essential role in the journey of overcoming Obsessive-Compulsive Disorder (OCD). Individuals suffering from OCD often experience isolation due to the nature of their compulsions and obsessions. Family and friends can provide a crucial support system that fosters understanding and compassion.

Their involvement can create a safe environment where individuals feel comfortable expressing their fears and struggles. This emotional support can significantly alleviate feelings of isolation and despair, making it easier for those affected to confront their challenges.

Educating family and friends about OCD is vital in helping them understand the disorder and its impact. Many people have misconceptions about OCD, often viewing it as merely a quirk or a preference for cleanliness. Providing information about the symptoms, triggers, and treatment options can help loved ones develop empathy and patience.

When family and friends are well-informed, they can better support the individual by recognizing the severity of their condition and encouraging them to seek professional help when necessary. Awareness can also guide them to respond appropriately during difficult moments, reducing frustration and confusion.

Encouragement from family and friends can motivate individuals to engage in treatment and practice coping strategies. The presence of supportive loved ones can encourage individuals to attend therapy sessions, adhere to treatment plans, and practice exposure and response prevention techniques. When family members participate in therapy sessions or learn about the treatment process, it fosters a collaborative approach to recovery.

This involvement can also help in addressing any relational dynamics that may contribute to the individual's OCD, allowing for healthier interactions and reducing triggers at home.

Setting boundaries is another significant aspect of how family and friends can assist someone with OCD. Loved ones must recognize the importance of allowing individuals to work through their compulsions and obsessions without inadvertently enabling them. By fostering a balance between support and independence, family and friends can help individuals take ownership of their recovery journey. This might involve setting limits on accommodating compulsions or encouraging healthier coping mechanisms. Establishing these boundaries helps prevent codependency and empowers individuals to confront their OCD more effectively.

Lastly, the emotional resilience of family and friends is crucial in dealing with the challenges that OCD presents. Supporting a loved one with OCD can be taxing, leading to feelings of frustration or helplessness. Family and friends must also prioritize their own mental health and seek support for themselves.

Engaging in support groups or therapy can help them process their feelings, learn effective communication strategies, and maintain their well-being. A healthy support system not only benefits the individual with OCD but also strengthens the bonds within the family or friendship circle, creating a nurturing environment conducive to healing.

Support Groups

Support groups play a vital role in the journey toward overcoming obsessive-compulsive disorder (OCD). These groups provide a safe and understanding environment where individuals can share their experiences, struggles, and successes. The collective knowledge and shared experiences among members can be invaluable, offering insights that may not be found in traditional therapy settings. By connecting with others who understand the unique challenges of OCD, participants often find a sense of belonging and validation that is crucial for healing.

Joining a support group can significantly reduce feelings of isolation that many people with OCD experience. When individuals hear others articulate their own obsessions and compulsions, it can be a powerful reminder that they are not alone in their struggles. This shared understanding fosters empathy and compassion, allowing members to express their feelings without fear of judgment. As members share coping strategies and personal anecdotes, they help one another see that recovery is possible and that there are various paths to finding peace.

In addition to emotional support, many support groups offer practical strategies for managing OCD symptoms. Facilitators or more experienced members often share techniques that have worked for them, such as exposure and response prevention (ERP) exercises or mindfulness practices. These strategies can complement the therapeutic techniques individuals are learning in their personal therapy sessions. Moreover, discussing these approaches within a group setting allows for immediate feedback and encouragement, which can enhance motivation and accountability.

Support groups can also serve as an educational resource. Many groups invite guest speakers, such as therapists or researchers, to discuss the latest findings and treatments for OCD. This access to expert knowledge can empower individuals with the tools and information they need to advocate for themselves in their treatment. Learning about the science behind OCD and its treatment options can demystify the disorder and help members feel more equipped to manage their symptoms effectively.

Finally, the duration of participation in a support group can vary based on individual needs. Some may find that they benefit from ongoing support for an extended period, while others may attend for a few months and then move on as they develop their coping strategies. Regardless of the length of involvement, the relationships formed within these groups can be lasting and impactful. By fostering connections and encouraging open dialogue, support groups provide a crucial component in the journey to overcoming OCD, helping individuals find solace, strength, and ultimately, peace.

Online Communities

Online communities have emerged as a vital resource for individuals seeking support in overcoming obsessive-compulsive disorder (OCD). These platforms provide a space where individuals can share their experiences, challenges, and successes in managing their symptoms. The anonymity afforded by the internet allows members to express their feelings without fear of judgment, fostering open and honest discussions about their struggles. This sense of connection can be particularly empowering for those who may feel isolated in their experiences.

One of the most significant advantages of online communities is the wealth of information they offer. Members often share valuable insights about various treatment options, coping strategies, and techniques they have found effective in managing OCD. From exposure and response prevention to mindfulness practices, the exchange of knowledge can help individuals discover new approaches to their recovery journey. Additionally, many communities feature resources such as articles, videos, and expert interviews that can further inform members about OCD and its treatment.

Support from peers in these communities can also play a crucial role in fostering resilience. When individuals share their stories, they often highlight the commonalities in their experiences, which can help others feel understood and less alone. Encouragement from fellow members can motivate individuals to stay committed to their treatment plans and implement new strategies. Celebrating small victories together can build a sense of camaraderie, reinforcing the importance of perseverance in overcoming OCD.

Furthermore, online communities often host discussions on various topics related to OCD, creating opportunities for members to learn from one another. These discussions may cover triggers, coping mechanisms, and the emotional toll of living with OCD. Engaging in these conversations allows individuals to gain different perspectives on their condition, helping them to develop a more comprehensive understanding of their symptoms and potential solutions. As members share their unique experiences, they contribute to a collective knowledge base that can benefit everyone involved.

Finally, while online communities can be tremendously beneficial, it is essential to approach them with a discerning mindset. Not all advice shared in these forums may be grounded in professional expertise, and individuals should be cautious about implementing suggestions without consulting a qualified mental health professional. Balancing peer support with expert guidance ensures a well-rounded approach to managing OCD. By leveraging the strengths of online communities while remaining vigilant about the quality of information shared, individuals can harness the power of collective support on their journey to overcoming OCD.

How To Overcome OCD

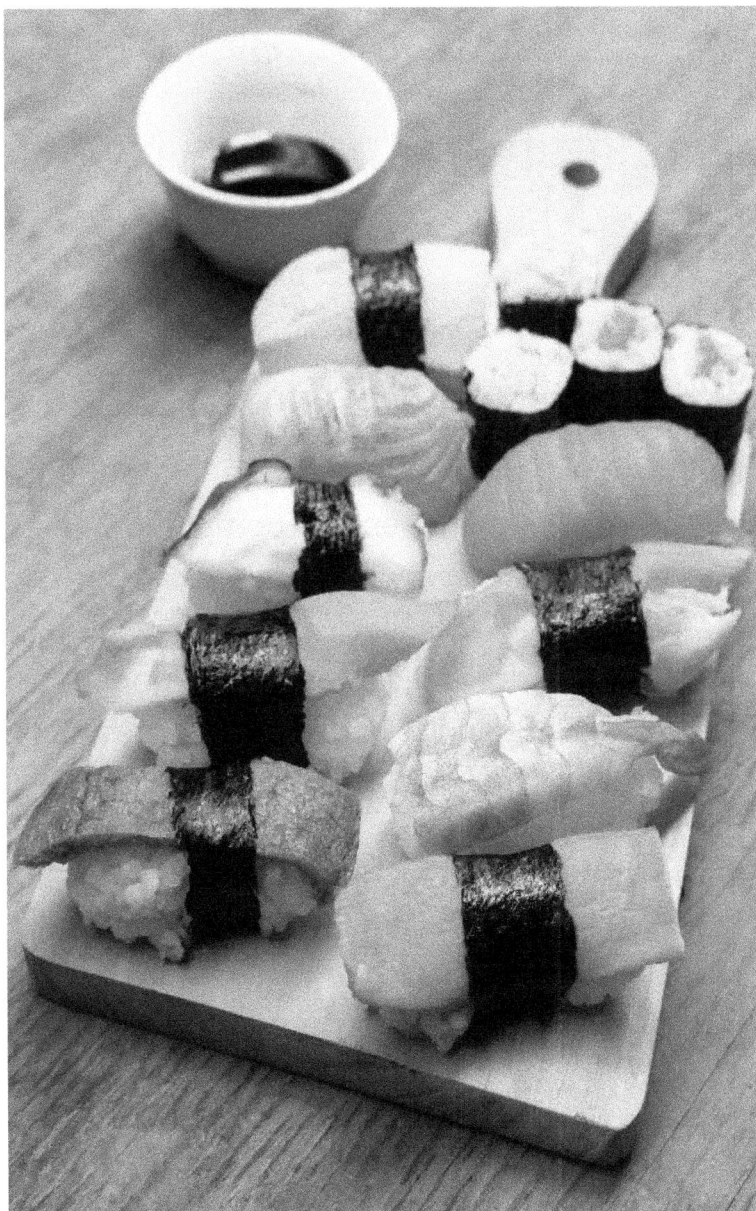

Chapter 8

Lifestyle Changes for Managing OCD

Nutrition and OCD

Nutrition plays a significant role in mental health, and its impact on obsessive-compulsive disorder (OCD) is gaining increased attention in recent years. The connection between diet and mental well-being is supported by emerging research that suggests certain nutrients can influence brain function and mood regulation.

For individuals dealing with OCD, adopting a balanced diet rich in essential vitamins and minerals may not only improve overall health but also help to alleviate some symptoms associated with the disorder.

One of the key nutrients important for brain health is omega-3 fatty acids, commonly found in fatty fish, flaxseeds, and walnuts. Omega-3s have been linked to reduced inflammation and improved neuronal function, which can be beneficial for individuals with OCD. Incorporating more omega-3-rich foods into one's diet may help enhance mood and cognitive function, potentially reducing the severity of obsessive thoughts and compulsive behaviors. Additionally, these fatty acids can promote overall cardiovascular health, which is crucial for maintaining a holistic approach to well-being.

Another vital component of a nutritious diet is the inclusion of whole grains, fruits, and vegetables. These foods are rich in fiber, vitamins, and antioxidants, which are essential for maintaining a healthy gut. Recent studies suggest a strong connection between gut health and mental health, highlighting the importance of the gut-brain axis. A balanced diet that supports gut health may contribute to a reduction in anxiety and depression symptoms, which often co-occur with OCD. Foods such as leafy greens, berries, and legumes can provide the necessary nutrients to support both physical and mental health.

Moreover, certain vitamins and minerals are particularly beneficial for those struggling with OCD. For example, magnesium, found in nuts, seeds, and leafy greens, has been shown to have a calming effect on the nervous system. Similarly, B vitamins, which can be obtained from whole grains, eggs, and dairy products, play a crucial role in energy production and can influence mood regulation. Ensuring adequate intake of these nutrients can support mental clarity and emotional stability, providing a solid foundation for individuals working to overcome OCD.

Finally, it is essential to consider the impact of sugar and processed foods on mental health. Diets high in refined sugars and unhealthy fats can lead to increased inflammation and mood swings, potentially exacerbating OCD symptoms. Reducing the consumption of these foods while focusing on whole, nutrient-dense options can lead to a more stable mood and improved mental clarity. For individuals looking to manage their OCD, making informed dietary choices can be a powerful strategy in their journey towards finding peace and stability.

Exercise and Mental Health

Exercise plays a critical role in mental health, particularly for individuals grappling with obsessive-compulsive disorder (OCD). Engaging in physical activity can lead to significant improvements in mood and overall psychological well-being. This is especially relevant for those with OCD, as the disorder often manifests with heightened anxiety and intrusive thoughts. Regular exercise can help to mitigate these symptoms by promoting the release of endorphins, which are natural mood lifters. Furthermore, the structured nature of a workout routine can provide a sense of control and accomplishment, countering the feelings of helplessness that often accompany OCD.

The physiological effects of exercise also contribute to mental health benefits. When individuals exercise, their bodies undergo various changes, including increased blood flow to the brain and enhanced neuroplasticity. These changes can lead to improved cognitive function, which is beneficial for those dealing with OCD. Enhanced cognitive function can help individuals better manage their thoughts and behaviors, making it easier to challenge obsessive thoughts and resist compulsions.

Additionally, specific forms of exercise, such as aerobic activities, have been shown to reduce anxiety levels, which can be particularly advantageous for someone struggling with the anxiety that often accompanies OCD.

Incorporating exercise into a daily routine can also foster a sense of community and social support, which is vital for mental health. Group activities, such as team sports or exercise classes, encourage social interaction and can alleviate feelings of isolation that many individuals with OCD experience. Building connections with others can provide additional emotional support, making it easier to navigate the challenges of OCD. Moreover, sharing experiences with others who understand similar struggles can create a sense of belonging, which can be incredibly therapeutic.

Mindfulness and relaxation techniques commonly associated with exercise can further benefit individuals with OCD. Practices such as yoga or tai chi combine physical movement with mindfulness, enabling participants to focus on their breath and body.

This mindfulness aspect can be particularly effective in helping individuals ground themselves in the present moment, reducing the tendency to become overwhelmed by intrusive thoughts. By integrating mindfulness into their exercise routine, individuals can develop healthier coping strategies, which can be instrumental in managing OCD symptoms.

Finally, it is essential for individuals with OCD to approach exercise in a balanced way. While physical activity can be a powerful tool for managing symptoms, over-exercising may lead to additional stress or anxiety. It is important to find a sustainable routine that fits individual preferences and lifestyles. Setting realistic goals and listening to the body's signals can help create a positive relationship with exercise.

By incorporating regular physical activity into their lives, individuals with OCD can take significant steps toward improving their mental health, ultimately contributing to a greater sense of peace and well-being.

Sleep Hygiene

Sleep hygiene refers to a set of practices and habits that are essential for promoting quality sleep. For individuals dealing with obsessive-compulsive disorder (OCD), maintaining good sleep hygiene can be particularly important, as poor sleep can exacerbate symptoms and reduce overall well-being. Establishing a consistent sleep routine, creating a comfortable sleep environment, and engaging in relaxation techniques can all contribute to better sleep quality, which in turn can help manage OCD symptoms more effectively.

One of the foundational aspects of sleep hygiene is maintaining a consistent sleep schedule. Going to bed and waking up at the same time every day helps regulate the body's internal clock, making it easier to fall asleep and wake up refreshed. For those with OCD, this consistency can also provide a sense of control and predictability, which can be comforting. It is advisable to limit naps during the day, as they can interfere with nighttime sleep, especially if taken too close to bedtime.

Creating a conducive sleep environment is another critical element of sleep hygiene. The bedroom should be a sanctuary for rest, free from distractions and disturbances. This includes keeping the room dark, quiet, and at a comfortable temperature. Investing in a good quality mattress and pillows that provide adequate support can also enhance sleep quality. For individuals with OCD, minimizing clutter in the bedroom may also reduce anxiety and promote a calming atmosphere, further aiding relaxation.

Establishing a pre-sleep routine can signal to the body that it is time to wind down. Engaging in calming activities such as reading, taking a warm bath, or practicing mindfulness meditation can help ease the transition to sleep. Limiting screen time in the hour leading up to bedtime is crucial, as the blue light emitted by devices can interfere with the production of melatonin, a hormone that regulates sleep. For those with OCD, incorporating cognitive-behavioral strategies during this time can also help in managing intrusive thoughts that may arise.

Finally, being mindful of dietary and lifestyle factors can significantly impact sleep hygiene. Avoiding caffeine and heavy meals close to bedtime can prevent disturbances in sleep patterns. Regular physical activity, when done at the right time, can also promote better sleep. While exercise is beneficial, it is best to avoid vigorous workouts in the evening, which may have an energizing effect. By prioritizing sleep hygiene, individuals with OCD can create a solid foundation for improving their overall mental health and managing their symptoms more effectively.

How To Overcome OCD

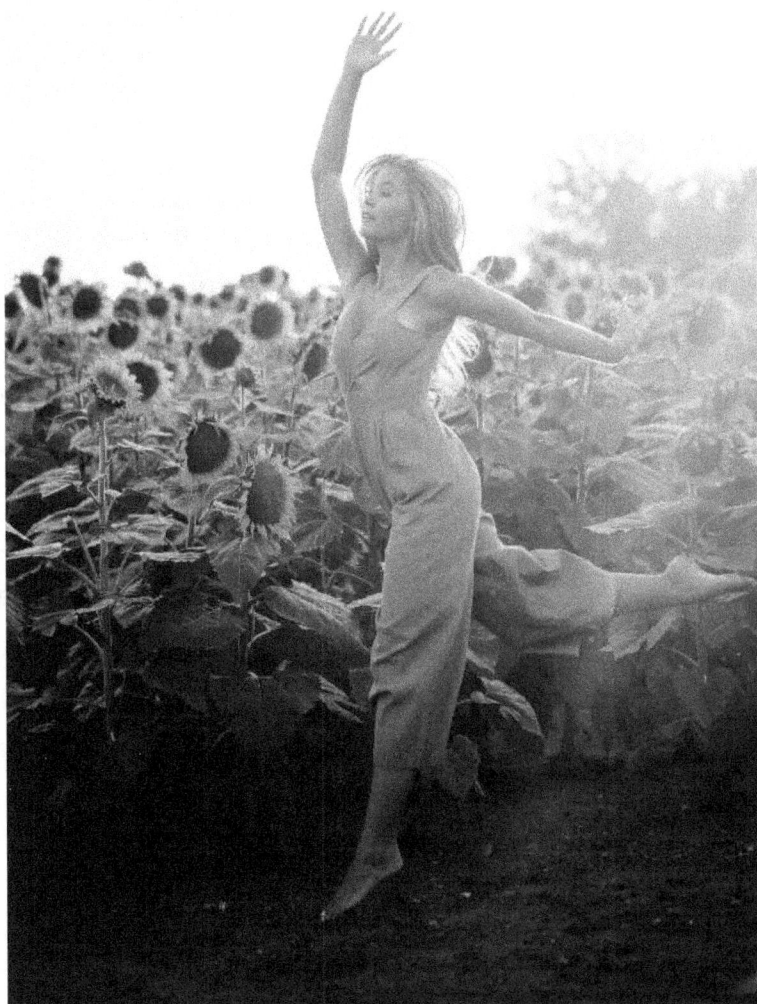

Strategies For Finding Peace

Chapter 9

Developing Coping Strategies

Journaling and Reflection

Journaling serves as a powerful tool for individuals seeking to understand and manage their obsessive-compulsive disorder (OCD). By committing thoughts and feelings to paper, individuals can create a safe space for exploring the complexities of their emotions and behaviors.

This practice allows for the externalization of internal struggles, making it easier to identify patterns and triggers associated with OCD. Regularly documenting experiences can lead to increased self-awareness and provide valuable insights into the nature of compulsions and obsessions.

In the process of journaling, it is essential to adopt an honest and non-judgmental approach. Writing freely without the fear of criticism fosters a sense of liberation, allowing individuals to articulate their fears and anxieties. This can be particularly beneficial for those with OCD, as it encourages them to confront their intrusive thoughts rather than suppressing them. By acknowledging these thoughts on paper, individuals can begin to dissect them analytically, distinguishing between reality and irrational fears. Over time, this practice can help diminish the power these thoughts hold, fostering a healthier mindset.

Reflection plays a crucial role in the journaling process. After writing, taking the time to reflect on what has been documented can lead to deeper understanding and personal growth. Individuals can ask themselves questions about the emotions behind their thoughts, the context in which they arise, and the effectiveness of their coping strategies. This reflective practice allows for the recognition of progress over time, highlighting moments of resilience and strength in the face of OCD. Regular reflection can also illuminate areas that require further attention or adjustment in one's coping strategies.

Incorporating structured prompts into journaling can enhance its effectiveness. Prompts may include questions like "What are my current triggers?" or "How did I respond to my OCD symptoms today?" These guided reflections can help maintain focus and provide direction, particularly during moments of heightened anxiety. Additionally, utilizing gratitude lists or positive affirmations within the journaling practice can help shift the focus from obsessive thoughts to more constructive and uplifting reflections. This shift not only promotes a sense of empowerment but also reinforces the idea that recovery is a journey filled with both challenges and victories.

Ultimately, journaling and reflection can be transformative for individuals grappling with OCD. By documenting their experiences and engaging in reflective practices, they can cultivate a deeper understanding of their condition. This self-awareness paves the way for more effective coping mechanisms and empowers individuals to take control of their narratives. As they navigate the complexities of OCD, journaling can serve as a steadfast companion, guiding them towards greater peace and resilience in their daily lives.

Distraction Techniques

Distraction techniques serve as valuable tools for individuals dealing with obsessive-compulsive disorder (OCD). These methods can help redirect focus away from intrusive thoughts and compulsive behaviors, providing a much-needed reprieve. Distraction can take many forms, from engaging in physical activities to immersing oneself in creative pursuits. The key is to find what resonates best with the individual, as preferences for distraction vary widely from person to person.

Physical activity is one of the most effective distraction techniques. Exercise releases endorphins, which can improve mood and reduce anxiety. Engaging in activities such as jogging, dancing, or even taking a brisk walk can help clear the mind and shift attention away from distressing thoughts. Additionally, the rhythmic nature of many physical activities can be meditative, allowing individuals to experience a state of flow where OCD symptoms may temporarily recede. Finding an enjoyable form of exercise can turn a necessary distraction into a pleasurable routine.

Creative pursuits also offer a powerful means of distraction. Activities such as painting, writing, or playing music not only engage the mind but also provide an outlet for emotions. These creative expressions can serve as a form of self-therapy, allowing individuals to process their feelings while diverting their attention from compulsive urges.

Setting aside time for creative endeavors can foster a sense of accomplishment and fulfillment, further aiding in the management of OCD symptoms.

Social engagement is another effective distraction technique. Interacting with friends, family, or support groups can provide emotional support and a sense of belonging.

Conversations and shared activities can help shift focus away from obsessive thoughts and reduce the isolation often felt by those with OCD. Whether it's participating in a group hobby, attending social events, or simply reaching out for a chat, building a supportive network can play a crucial role in maintaining mental well-being.

Finally, mindfulness practices can complement distraction techniques by promoting awareness of the present moment. Techniques such as deep breathing, meditation, or yoga can help ground individuals, making it easier to let go of intrusive thoughts. While mindfulness itself is not a distraction in the traditional sense, it can create a mental space where distractions can be more readily embraced. By combining mindfulness with other distraction techniques, individuals can develop a comprehensive strategy for overcoming OCD and finding peace.

Positive Affirmations

Positive affirmations are powerful tools that can significantly contribute to the management of Obsessive-Compulsive Disorder (OCD). These short, positive statements help counteract negative thought patterns that often accompany OCD. By consistently repeating affirmations, individuals can reshape their mindset, reduce anxiety, and foster a more positive self-image. This practice encourages a shift in focus from intrusive thoughts and compulsive behaviors to self-empowerment and resilience.

To effectively incorporate positive affirmations into your daily routine, it is essential to identify specific areas of concern related to your OCD. Begin by reflecting on the thoughts and fears that trigger your compulsions. Once you have a clearer understanding of these triggers, you can craft personalized affirmations that address these specific issues. For example, if you struggle with fears of contamination, an affirmation like "I am safe and in control" can serve as a powerful reminder of your strength and capability to manage your anxiety.

Repetition is key to the effectiveness of positive affirmations. It is advisable to practice them daily, ideally in the morning and before bed. This consistency helps to reinforce the positive messages in your subconscious mind. Many find it helpful to write their affirmations down and place them in visible locations, such as mirrors or workspaces, to serve as constant reminders throughout the day.

Additionally, combining affirmations with mindfulness exercises can enhance their impact, allowing individuals to ground themselves in the present moment while affirming their strength.

As you begin to integrate positive affirmations into your life, it is important to approach this practice with patience and an open mind. Change may not occur immediately, and it is natural to face challenges along the way. However, with regular practice, you are likely to notice gradual shifts in your thought patterns and emotional responses. Over time, affirmations can help reduce the intensity of OCD symptoms, enabling you to navigate daily challenges with greater ease and confidence.

Lastly, remember that positive affirmations are just one component of a comprehensive approach to managing OCD. While they can be effective in promoting a positive mindset, they work best when combined with other strategies such as cognitive-behavioral therapy, exposure and response prevention, and support groups. By incorporating positive affirmations alongside these methods, you can create a well-rounded approach to overcoming OCD and achieving a sense of peace in your life.

How To Overcome OCD

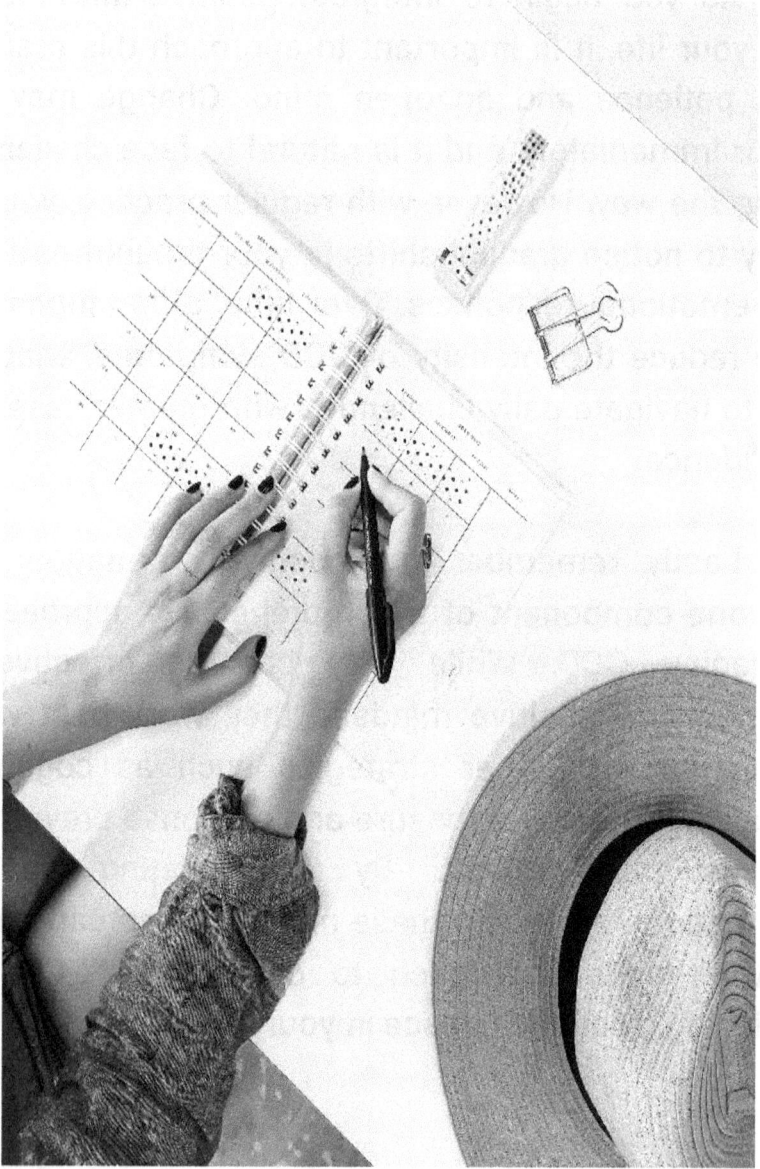

Chapter 10

Long-Term Management of OCD

Setting Realistic Goals

Setting realistic goals is a crucial step in the journey to overcoming obsessive-compulsive disorder (OCD). Many individuals with OCD may have a tendency to set overly ambitious or unrealistic goals, which can lead to feelings of frustration and disappointment. To effectively manage OCD, it is essential to establish goals that are attainable and measurable. This not only helps in building confidence but also facilitates gradual progress in facing the challenges associated with OCD.

When setting realistic goals, it is important to break down larger objectives into smaller, manageable tasks. For instance, instead of aiming to completely eliminate all compulsive behaviors overnight, individuals can focus on reducing the frequency of specific rituals over a designated period.

By setting small, incremental goals, individuals can celebrate their achievements along the way, which reinforces positive behavior and boosts motivation. This stepwise approach allows for a more sustainable and less overwhelming path towards recovery.

Another key aspect of goal-setting is ensuring that the goals are specific and time-bound. Vague goals can lead to ambiguity and a lack of direction, which may contribute to anxiety. Instead of stating, "I want to feel better," a more effective goal would be, "I will practice exposure therapy for ten minutes every day for the next two weeks." This specificity not only clarifies what needs to be done but also provides a timeline for accountability. Tracking progress against these specific goals can help individuals recognize their advancements, even if they are small.

In addition to specificity and manageability, it is vital to remain flexible in goal-setting. OCD can be unpredictable, and there may be days when progress feels stalled or setbacks occur. It is important for individuals to acknowledge that this is a natural part of the recovery process.

Goals should be revisited and adjusted as necessary, allowing for a level of adaptability that accommodates fluctuations in motivation and circumstances. This flexibility can prevent feelings of failure when things do not go as planned and foster resilience in the face of challenges.

Finally, seeking support from mental health professionals or support groups can enhance the goal-setting process. Engaging with therapists who specialize in OCD can provide valuable insights into what constitutes realistic goals based on individual circumstances.

Additionally, sharing goals with supportive friends or family members can create a sense of accountability and encouragement. By collaborating with others and utilizing available resources, individuals can set themselves up for success in their journey to overcome OCD, ultimately leading to a more peaceful and fulfilling life.

Monitoring Progress

Monitoring progress in the journey to overcome OCD is a vital aspect of the recovery process. This involves not only tracking symptoms but also observing changes in behavior, thoughts, and overall emotional well-being.

By establishing a clear framework for monitoring, individuals can gain insights into their triggers, responses, and the effectiveness of various strategies employed to manage OCD. Regular assessment helps to identify patterns and areas that may require additional focus, ensuring that the path to recovery remains constructive and tailored to personal needs.

One practical approach to monitoring progress is the use of journaling. Keeping a daily or weekly log of thoughts, feelings, and behaviors can provide valuable data for self-reflection. Individuals can note specific instances of OCD symptoms, their intensity, and the circumstances surrounding them.

Additionally, recording coping strategies used in response to these symptoms can help to evaluate their effectiveness over time. This practice encourages accountability and enables individuals to celebrate small victories, reinforcing positive changes in their mindset and behavior.

Another effective method for tracking progress is through regular check-ins with a therapist or support group. Engaging in discussions about experiences, challenges, and achievements fosters a sense of community and understanding.

A professional can offer objective feedback, helping to identify areas of improvement and suggesting adjustments to current strategies. These interactions also provide opportunities to learn from others' experiences, which can be inspiring and motivating. Open communication is essential for maintaining momentum in the recovery process.

Setting measurable goals is another crucial aspect of monitoring progress. By establishing specific, achievable objectives, individuals can create a roadmap that outlines desired outcomes.

These goals may include reducing the frequency of compulsive behaviors, minimizing anxiety levels in specific situations, or increasing engagement in enjoyable activities. Reviewing and adjusting these goals periodically ensures that they remain relevant and attainable, providing a clear sense of direction and purpose in the ongoing battle against OCD.

Lastly, it is important to acknowledge that progress may not always be linear. Individuals may experience setbacks or periods of heightened anxiety despite their efforts. Recognizing that this is a normal part of the recovery journey is essential for maintaining motivation and resilience.

Emphasizing the importance of self-compassion during these times can help individuals stay focused on their long-term goals. By monitoring progress thoughtfully and consistently, individuals can equip themselves with the tools needed to navigate the complexities of OCD and ultimately find peace.

Maintaining Peace

Maintaining peace while managing Obsessive-Compulsive Disorder (OCD) is a crucial aspect of the journey toward recovery. Individuals with OCD often experience intrusive thoughts and compulsive behaviors that can disrupt their sense of tranquility. To combat these challenges, it is essential to develop strategies that foster a peaceful mindset. This involves understanding the nature of OCD, establishing healthy routines, and incorporating mindfulness practices into daily life.

Understanding the triggers of OCD is the first step in maintaining peace. Each person with OCD may have unique triggers, whether they relate to cleanliness, order, or more abstract concerns. By identifying these triggers, individuals can work to minimize their exposure and develop coping mechanisms. This may involve keeping a journal to track thoughts and feelings related to OCD, which can provide insights into patterns and help in recognizing when to employ specific strategies to regain peace.

Establishing a consistent daily routine is another effective strategy for maintaining peace. Routines create a sense of predictability and control, which can be particularly beneficial for those with OCD. Incorporating structured time for relaxation, exercise, and hobbies can also provide a balanced lifestyle that counters the anxiety often associated with OCD. By prioritizing self-care and ensuring that there is time for activities that bring joy, individuals can cultivate a more peaceful existence.

Mindfulness and meditation practices can significantly enhance one's ability to maintain peace. These practices encourage individuals to focus on the present moment, reducing the power of intrusive thoughts.

Techniques such as deep breathing, guided imagery, or body scans can help ground individuals during times of heightened anxiety. Regular practice of mindfulness can create a mental space where individuals feel less overwhelmed by OCD, allowing for greater emotional regulation and a sense of calm.

Lastly, seeking support from professionals and peers can play a vital role in maintaining peace. Therapy options such as Cognitive Behavioral Therapy (CBT) specifically target the symptoms of OCD and provide tools for coping. Support groups can also offer a sense of community and understanding, reminding individuals that they are not alone in their struggles. Sharing experiences and strategies with others who face similar challenges can foster resilience and reinforce the peace that individuals seek on their journey to overcoming OCD.

How To Overcome OCD

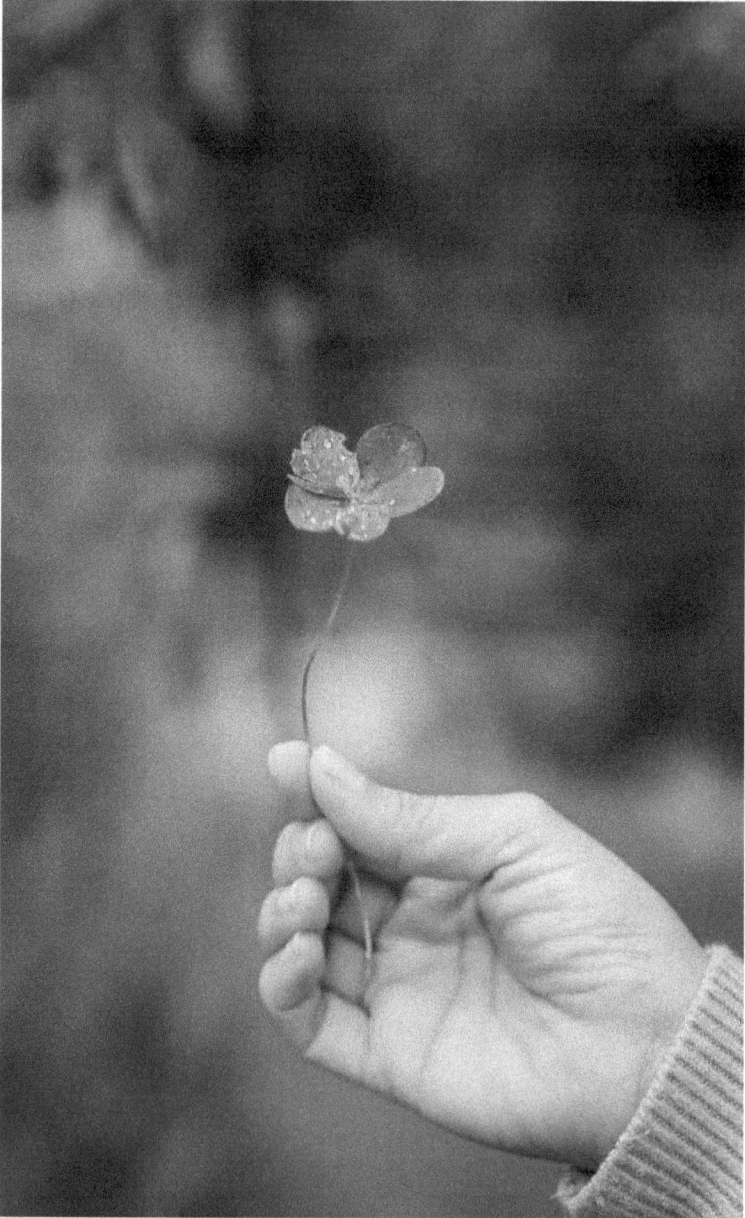

Chapter 11

Success Stories and Testimonials

Personal Accounts of Overcoming OCD

Personal accounts of individuals who have successfully navigated the challenges of obsessive-compulsive disorder (OCD) provide valuable insights and inspiration for those currently struggling. These stories often highlight the diverse nature of OCD and the various strategies employed to combat its hold. Each account serves as a reminder that recovery is possible and that personal experiences can offer guidance and hope to others on a similar path.

One individual, Emily, describes her journey through the labyrinth of OCD, characterized by intrusive thoughts and compulsive behaviors that dominated her daily life. She recounts how her turning point came when she recognized the need for professional help.

By seeking therapy, Emily learned about exposure and response prevention (ERP), a technique that gradually exposed her to her fears while preventing her from resorting to compulsions. This process was daunting, but through persistence and support from her therapist, she began to reclaim her life, finding strength in confronting her fears rather than succumbing to them.

Another powerful narrative comes from Mark, who dealt with contamination fears that dictated his every action. Mark shares how he implemented a combination of cognitive-behavioral therapy (CBT) and mindfulness practices. By challenging irrational thoughts and accepting uncertainty, he gradually reduced the power of his compulsions. His daily practice of mindfulness not only helped him stay grounded during moments of anxiety but also fostered a greater acceptance of his thoughts, allowing them to pass without judgment. Mark emphasizes the importance of patience and self-compassion, noting that progress is often nonlinear but still achievable.

Sophia's experience highlights the significance of community support in overcoming OCD. After years of battling her symptoms in isolation, she joined a support group where she met others facing similar struggles. Sharing her story and hearing others' experiences helped her feel less alone and provided her with new strategies for coping.

The group dynamic offered a safe space for vulnerability, enabling Sophia to confront her fears while receiving encouragement and accountability from peers who understood her journey. This sense of belonging became a crucial component of her recovery process.

Finally, David's account illustrates the role of lifestyle changes in managing OCD. He discovered that incorporating regular exercise, a balanced diet, and adequate sleep significantly impacted his mental health. By prioritizing self-care, David found that his resilience against obsessive thoughts improved. He also began journaling as a way to process his emotions and track his progress.

Through these lifestyle adjustments and ongoing therapy, David learned that recovery is not only about confronting compulsions but also about nurturing overall well-being. His story serves as a reminder that a holistic approach can complement traditional treatments in the journey toward overcoming OCD.

Lessons Learned

Overcoming Obsessive-Compulsive Disorder (OCD) is a journey that often involves a steep learning curve. Individuals grappling with OCD frequently discover that their experiences teach them valuable lessons about themselves, their triggers, and the nature of their compulsions. One primary lesson learned is the importance of self-awareness. Being able to identify specific thoughts, feelings, and situations that provoke obsessive thinking or compulsive behavior allows individuals to develop better coping strategies. Self-awareness acts as a foundation for implementing practical techniques that can reduce the intensity of OCD symptoms.

Another significant lesson is the power of community and support. Many people underestimate the benefits of connecting with others who share similar struggles. Support groups and therapy sessions provide a safe space for individuals to share their experiences and feelings. By engaging with others, individuals learn that they are not alone in their battle. This sense of community fosters encouragement and accountability, reminding them that recovery is not solely an individual effort but can also be a collective journey.

Cognitive Behavioral Therapy (CBT) is often highlighted as a crucial tool in overcoming OCD, and many have learned that the strategies it offers are not just temporary fixes but lifelong skills. The lessons derived from CBT, such as exposure and response prevention (ERP), emphasize gradual exposure to anxiety-inducing stimuli while refraining from compulsive behaviors. This process teaches individuals that they can tolerate discomfort and that the anxiety associated with their obsessions will diminish over time. Mastering these skills can lead to increased confidence in handling future challenges.

Mindfulness practices have also emerged as a vital lesson in managing OCD. Many individuals have found that incorporating mindfulness techniques, such as meditation and deep-breathing exercises, can significantly reduce anxiety levels and enhance overall mental well-being. These practices encourage individuals to stay present and acknowledge their thoughts without judgment, ultimately allowing them to break the cycle of obsessive thinking. The realization that they can cultivate a sense of peace amidst the chaos of OCD has been transformative for many.

Lastly, individuals often learn the importance of patience and self-compassion throughout their journey. Overcoming OCD is rarely a linear process; setbacks are common and can be disheartening. Recognizing that recovery takes time and allowing oneself to experience the full range of emotions without self-criticism is crucial. This understanding fosters a more forgiving attitude towards oneself, encouraging persistence in the face of challenges. Embracing patience and self-compassion not only aids in managing OCD but also enriches one's overall mental health and resilience.

Hope for the Future

The journey toward overcoming obsessive-compulsive disorder (OCD) can often feel overwhelming and isolating. However, it is essential to recognize that there is hope for the future. Many individuals diagnosed with OCD have successfully navigated their way to a more peaceful and fulfilling life. This transformation is achievable through a combination of therapeutic strategies, support systems, and personal resilience. By focusing on the possibility of recovery, individuals can cultivate a more positive mindset that fosters healing and growth.

One of the most effective strategies for managing OCD is cognitive-behavioral therapy (CBT), particularly exposure and response prevention (ERP). This therapeutic approach helps individuals confront their fears gradually while learning to resist the compulsive behaviors that often accompany these fears. Research consistently demonstrates that CBT and ERP are highly effective in reducing OCD symptoms. By committing to this therapeutic process, individuals can reclaim control over their thoughts and behaviors, leading to significant improvements in their quality of life.

In addition to professional therapy, support from family, friends, and support groups can provide a vital lifeline for those dealing with OCD. Connecting with others who understand the challenges of OCD can foster a sense of belonging and reduce feelings of isolation. Support groups, whether in-person or online, allow individuals to share their experiences, tips, and coping mechanisms. This communal aspect of recovery can reinforce the notion that one is not alone in their struggles, instilling hope and encouragement for the future.

Mindfulness and self-care practices also play a crucial role in managing OCD symptoms. Techniques such as meditation, yoga, and journaling can help individuals develop a greater awareness of their thoughts and feelings, creating space for acceptance and self-compassion. By incorporating these practices into daily routines, individuals can cultivate resilience, reduce stress, and improve their overall mental health. This holistic approach not only aids in managing OCD but also enhances emotional well-being, paving the way for a brighter future.

Ultimately, the future holds immense potential for individuals battling OCD. By embracing effective treatment options, seeking support, and prioritizing self-care, it is possible to break free from the constraints of OCD. The journey may be challenging, but with determination and the right strategies, individuals can find peace and fulfillment in their lives. Hope is not just an abstract concept; it is a tangible force that can propel individuals toward recovery and a life enriched with possibility.

How To Overcome OCD

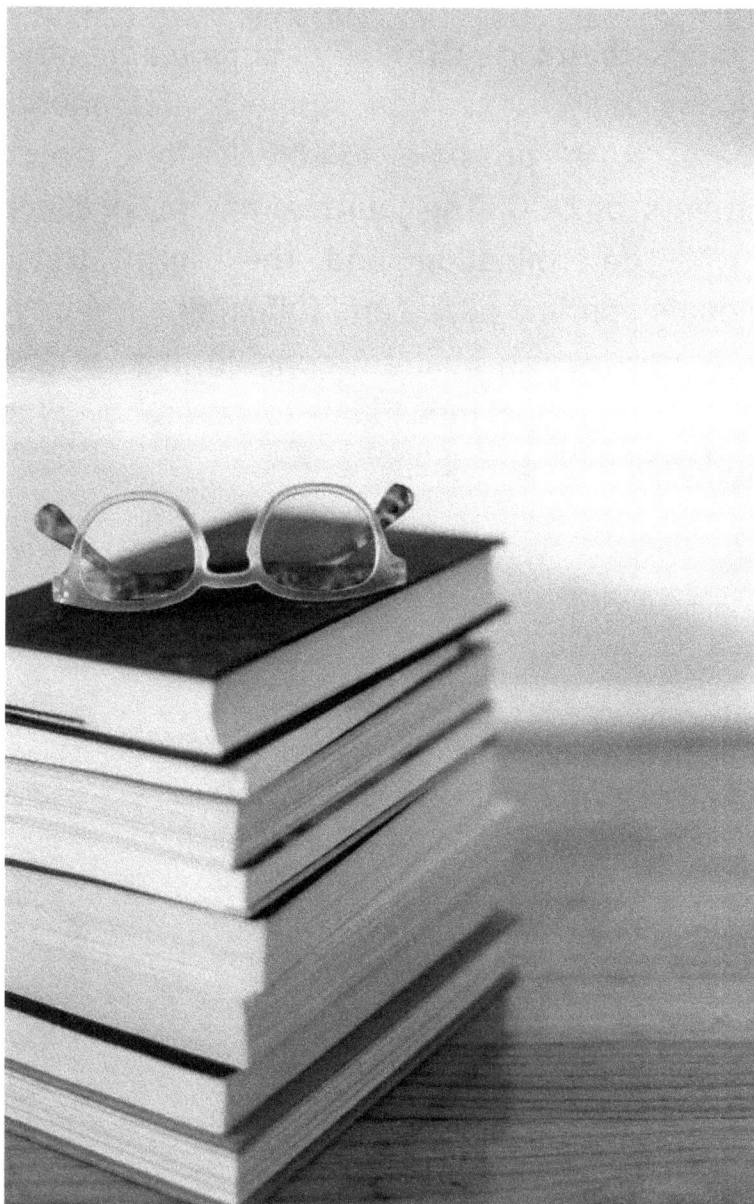

Chapter 12

Resources and Further Reading

Recommended Books

In the journey to overcome Obsessive-Compulsive Disorder (OCD), literature can serve as a powerful tool for understanding and managing symptoms. Several books provide insights into the condition, offering practical strategies and personal anecdotes that resonate with those experiencing OCD. These recommended readings can enhance knowledge, provide comfort, and inspire hope, making them valuable resources for anyone seeking to navigate their OCD challenges.

One highly regarded book is "The OCD Workbook: Your Guide to Breaking Free from Obsessive-Compulsive Disorder." This practical workbook combines cognitive-behavioral therapy techniques with exercises designed to help individuals confront their compulsions and obsessions.

The authors guide readers through step-by-step processes, enabling them to identify triggers and develop coping strategies. By actively engaging with the material, readers can gain a better understanding of their OCD and learn effective methods to reduce its impact on their daily lives.

Another essential read is "Brain Lock: Free Yourself from Obsessive-Compulsive Behavior." In this book, Dr. Jeffrey Schwartz introduces a four-step method that empowers individuals to take control of their thoughts and behaviors. Through a blend of neuroscience and personal stories, Schwartz illustrates how the brain can be rewired to combat OCD.

His approach emphasizes the importance of mindfulness and self-awareness in overcoming compulsive behaviors, making this a crucial resource for those looking for a structured plan to tackle their OCD.

For those interested in personal narratives, "The Boy Who Couldn't Stop Washing" by Judith L. Rappaport offers a compelling account of one family's experience with OCD. This book provides insight into the emotional and psychological toll that OCD can take on individuals and their loved ones. Rappaport's storytelling not only sheds light on the disorder but also highlights the resilience and strength found in the struggle against OCD. Readers can find solace in knowing they are not alone, and the shared experiences may inspire them to seek help and pursue recovery.

Lastly, "Freedom from Obsessive-Compulsive Disorder: A Personalized Recovery Program for Living with Uncertainty" by Jonathan Grayson is an invaluable resource for those looking to develop a personalized approach to managing OCD. Grayson emphasizes the importance of addressing the unique aspects of each individual's experience with OCD, offering tools to create a tailored recovery plan. By focusing on embracing uncertainty and challenging avoidance behaviors, this book empowers readers to take actionable steps toward reclaiming their lives from OCD.

Incorporating these recommended books into one's journey can provide essential support and guidance. They not only offer practical strategies and insights but also foster a sense of community and understanding among those affected by OCD. By engaging with these texts, individuals can equip themselves with the knowledge and tools necessary to confront their challenges and move toward a more peaceful existence.

Websites and Online Tools

Websites and online tools can serve as valuable resources for individuals seeking to overcome Obsessive-Compulsive Disorder (OCD). The internet provides a wealth of information, support networks, and therapeutic resources that can help individuals manage their symptoms. Many reputable organizations, such as the International OCD Foundation (IOCDF) and the Anxiety and Depression Association of America (ADAA), offer extensive information on OCD, including treatment options, self-help strategies, and the latest research. These websites often feature articles, blogs, and videos that explain OCD in detail, helping individuals understand their condition better and feel less isolated.

Online forums and support groups can be particularly beneficial for those dealing with OCD. Websites like Reddit and Facebook host communities where individuals can connect with others who share similar experiences. These platforms allow users to share their stories, seek advice, and provide support to one another. This sense of community can be comforting and empowering, as it reminds individuals that they are not alone in their struggles. Engaging with others who understand the challenges of OCD can foster a sense of belonging and motivate individuals to take proactive steps toward recovery.

In addition to community support, numerous online tools can aid in the management of OCD symptoms. Mobile applications such as "OCD Coach" and "nOCD" provide users with strategies and exercises based on cognitive-behavioral therapy (CBT) principles. These apps often include features like mood tracking, exposure exercises, and guided meditations, enabling users to practice coping skills in their daily lives. Incorporating these tools into a regular routine can enhance self-awareness and provide immediate support when faced with anxiety-provoking situations.

Telehealth services have also become a significant resource for individuals seeking professional help for OCD. Many therapists now offer online therapy sessions, allowing individuals to access treatment from the comfort of their homes. This can be particularly advantageous for those who may feel overwhelmed by the prospect of attending in-person appointments. Online therapy can provide flexibility in scheduling and eliminate travel barriers, making it easier for individuals to seek help and stay committed to their treatment plans.

Lastly, educational webinars and online workshops hosted by mental health professionals offer an opportunity for individuals to learn more about OCD and effective coping strategies. These sessions often cover a range of topics, from understanding the science behind OCD to practical techniques for managing intrusive thoughts. Participating in these events can empower individuals with knowledge and skills that are essential for their journey toward overcoming OCD. By leveraging these websites and online tools, individuals can create a comprehensive support system that aids in their pursuit of peace and recovery.

Professional Organizations

Professional organizations dedicated to the field of mental health, particularly those focusing on obsessive-compulsive disorder (OCD), play a crucial role in providing resources, support, and education for individuals seeking to overcome their challenges. These organizations often serve as a bridge between research, clinical practice, and the general public, ensuring that the latest findings and effective strategies are readily accessible. By engaging with these organizations, individuals can gain valuable insights into OCD, learn about treatment options, and find communities of support that can make a significant difference in their journey toward recovery.

One of the most prominent organizations is the International OCD Foundation (IOCDF), which focuses on raising awareness and promoting effective treatment for OCD. The IOCDF offers a wealth of resources, including educational materials, online forums, and directories of treatment providers. They also host annual conferences that bring together professionals and individuals affected by OCD, fostering an environment of learning and sharing.

By participating in these events, individuals can connect with others facing similar challenges and discover new coping strategies and treatment modalities.

Another important organization is the Anxiety and Depression Association of America (ADAA), which provides resources not only for OCD but also for related anxiety disorders. The ADAA emphasizes the importance of evidence-based treatments and offers a variety of online resources, including webinars, articles, and self-help tools. Their commitment to education and support empowers individuals to take an active role in their recovery, helping them to understand the nature of their condition and the various therapeutic options available. Engaging with the ADAA can also help individuals stay informed about the latest research developments and treatment trends.

Local support groups, often organized by professional organizations, can also be invaluable. These groups create safe spaces for individuals to share their experiences, challenges, and successes in managing OCD.

Many organizations facilitate these gatherings, either in-person or online, allowing participants to connect with others who truly understand their struggles. Being part of a supportive community can alleviate feelings of isolation and provide encouragement, making the journey towards overcoming OCD feel less daunting.

In addition to direct support and resources, professional organizations often advocate for public policy changes and increased funding for mental health research. By supporting these initiatives, individuals can contribute to a broader movement that seeks to improve treatment access and quality for all those affected by OCD. Becoming involved with professional organizations not only enhances personal recovery efforts but also fosters a collective push toward a better understanding and management of OCD at a societal level.

Author Notes & Acknowledgments

First and foremost, I would like to express my deepest gratitude to the people who inspired and supported me throughout the journey of writing this book. This project would not have been possible without their unwavering belief in me and their invaluable contributions.

To my wife, thank you for your constant encouragement and understanding. Your love and support have been my anchor during the challenging times of researching and writing this book. Your belief in my ability to make a difference in people's lives has been my driving force.

I would also like to disclose that this book contains some renewed artificial intelligence-generated content. I really appreciate very recent technological innovation by outstanding scientists and of course our reader's understanding.

Lastly, I want to express my deepest gratitude to the readers of this book. I sincerely hope the strategies and methods outlined within these pages will provide you with the knowledge and tools needed to truly make your life much better. Your commitment to seeking any good solutions and willingness to explore multiple methods is commendable.

Author Bio

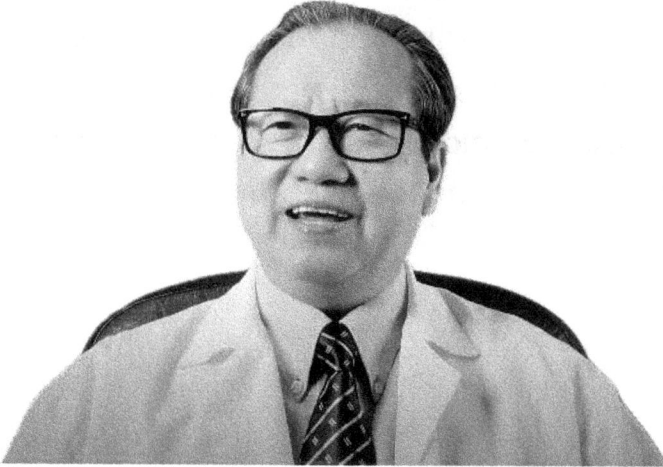

Johnson Wu earned his MD in 1982. With over 40 years of clinical experience, he has worked in hospitals in Zhejiang and Shanghai, China, as well as the Royal Marsden Hospital (part of Imperial College) in London, UK. Upon the recommendation of Sir Aaron Klug, the president of The Royal Society and a Nobel Prize winner in Chemistry, Dr. Wu was honorably awarded a British Royal Society Fellowship. He has published over 100 medical books in many countries and currently practices medicine in Canada.